# Back Pain

## By

## DR. Keith Smigiel NP, DC

Copyright © 2020 by DR. Keith Smigiel NP, DC

All rights reserved. No part of this book may be reproduced in any form, whether electronic or mechanical means, or be used in any manner without the expressed written permission of the copyright owner, except for the use of quotations in book reviews.

Printed in the Unites States of America

First Printing, 2020

ISBN- 9798619387971

# TABLE OF CONTENTS

**CHAPTER 1** *HOW ONE EVENT AND ONE DISCUSSION CHANGED THE COURSE OF MY LIFE* .................................................................................. 1

**CHAPTER 2** *A BIT OF ANATOMY: UNDERSTANDING THE BACK AND WHY IT IS SO EASY TO INJURE* ................................................................ 20

THE SPINE – AN OVERVIEW ................................................................ 22
THE MUSCLES ....................................................................................... 23
THE SPINE ............................................................................................. 25
THE NERVES ......................................................................................... 28
WHY BACKS ARE SO EASY TO INJURY ................................................ 31

**CHAPTER 3** *MECHANICS OF BACK INJURY, DIFFERENT PAIN DRIVERS OF LOW BACK PAIN* ..................................................................................... 34

DIFFERENT TYPES OF PAIN .................................................................. 35
YOUR BODY AND PAIN ........................................................................ 35
UNDERSTANDING YOUR BACK PAIN .................................................. 39
WHEN IT ISN'T MECHANICAL .............................................................. 43
RISK FACTORS ...................................................................................... 44
COMMON CAUSES – YOUR BACK'S HISTORY ................................... 49
GENETICS .............................................................................................. 50
EVERY DAY WEAR ................................................................................ 53

INJURIES ............................................................................................... 57

## CHAPTER 4 *TYPES OF INJURIES* ........................................................ 59

COMMON CAUSES OF INJURY ............................................................. 62
   ACUTE INJURIES ................................................................................. 64
   OVERUSE OR REPETITIVE INJURIES ...................................................... 66
   WHEN TO SEE A MEDICAL PROFESSIONAL ........................................... 68
POST-SURGERY ..................................................................................... 69
   SURGERY CONSIDERATIONS ............................................................... 69
   QUICK TEST ........................................................................................ 72
CHRONIC PAIN ...................................................................................... 74

## CHAPTER 5 *WHAT MEDICINE HAS TO OFFER* .................................. 78

THE DIFFERENT KINDS OF BACK PAIN MEDICATIONS ......................... 80
   NSAIDS ............................................................................................... 81
   MUSCLE RELAXERS ............................................................................. 82
   OPIOIDS .............................................................................................. 83
   ANTIDEPRESSANTS .............................................................................. 83
THE GOOD ............................................................................................ 85
THE BAD ............................................................................................... 86
MEDICATION ADDICTION AND RELIANCE ........................................... 89
HOW I HELP WEAN PATIENTS AWAY FROM A RELIANCE ON MEDICINE ............ 91

## CHAPTER 6 *TRAUMA, MENTAL HEALTH, AND THE OPIOID CRISIS* ....... 93

A BRIEF HISTORY – HOW WE GOT HERE ............................................. 95
MANAGING CHRONIC PAIN ................................................................. 98
TREATING A SYMPTOM – NOT THE PROBLEM .................................. 100

THE ROLE OF MENTAL HEALTH IN RECOVERY - *ANGELA* SMIGIEL, *MSW*, *LCSW* .................................................................................................... 103
EYE MOVEMENT DESENSITIZATION AND REPROCESSING ................................. 111
COGNITIVE BEHAVIORAL THERAPY .............................................................. 113

The Connection between Mental Health, Chronic Pain, and the Opioid Epidemic    117

## CHAPTER 7 *OLD SCHOOL VERSUS NEW SCHOOL TREATMENT FOR PAIN* .................................................................................................... 118

MECHANICAL BACK PAIN VS INFLAMMATORY ........................................... 120
IDENTIFYING THE PAIN DRIVER ................................................................ 123
PRIMARY PAIN DRIVER ............................................................................ 126
SECONDARY PAIN DRIVER ....................................................................... 127
TREATMENT FOR DRIVERS ...................................................................... 129
TYPES OF PAIN DRIVER ASSESSMENTS .................................................... 130
FUNCTIONAL BLOOD LAB ANALYSIS ........................................................ 131
DYNAMIC ULTRASOUND ASSESSMENT .................................................... 134
GAIT ANALYSIS ...................................................................................... 136
USING THE RIGHT TOOLS TO SOLVE THE PROBLEM .................................. 138

## CHAPTER 8 *BREAKING THE PAIN CYCLE* ............................................ 139

UNDERSTANDING THE CAUSE .................................................................. 141
THE DIFFERENCE BETWEEN PAIN AND DAMAGE ....................................... 144
AN APPREHENSIVE ANTICIPATION OF PAIN ............................................... 146
LEVELS OF PAIN ..................................................................................... 147

## CHAPTER 9 *START HEALING YOUR LOWER BACK TODAY* ................. 149

| | |
|---|---|
| **IMMEDIATE ACTION** | **151** |
| COLD AND HOT | 152 |
| UPDATE YOUR WORK SPACE | 153 |
| START CHANGING YOUR DIET AND EXERCISE ROUTINE | 156 |
| BETTER SLEEP | 157 |
| LOOK AT YOUR OTHER OPTIONS | 157 |
| **PLANNING FOR THE FUTURE** | **159** |
| PREVENTATIVE MEASURES TO KEEP YOUR BACK HEALTHY | 160 |
| ENDORPHINS – A NATURAL PAIN RELIEVER | 161 |
| **ONE DAY AT A TIME** | **163** |

## CHAPTER 10 *YOU ARE IN CHARGE* ............ 166

| | |
|---|---|
| **JOURNALS THAT MAY HELP** | **168** |
| PAIN JOURNAL | 169 |
| DIET JOURNAL | 170 |
| EXERCISE JOURNAL | 170 |
| **CORRECT MOTIONS TO REDUCE STRESS AND LOADS TO YOUR BACK** | **172** |
| HIP HINGE | 173 |
| LIFTING | 174 |
| GETTING DRESSED | 175 |
| GAIT ANALYSIS | 176 |
| **EXERCISES TO HELP YOU BE KINDER TO YOUR BACK** | **179** |
| GLUTEUS MEDIAS ACTIVATION | 180 |
| PIRIFORMIS STRETCH | 181 |
| CORE STABILITY – PELVIC TILT | 182 |
| PELVIC TILT | 182 |
| THE BIRD DOG | 183 |
| MEDITATION | 183 |
| **ESTABLISHING A ROUTINE** | **184** |
| **PHYSICAL THERAPY** | **186** |

**CHAPTER 11 *OTHER JOINTS* ............................................................ 189**

**BENEFITS BEYOND THE BACK**.................................................................. 191
**HOW YOUR WHOLE BODY CAN BENEFIT**.................................................. 193
**MIND OVER MEDICINE** ............................................................................ 197

# CHAPTER 1

# How One Event and One Discussion Changed the Course of My Life

Ever since I can remember I have always had an innate curiosity about how things work or the underlying mechanics of things. My mother tells stories of finding me with her appliances and telephones taken apart and I would enjoy putting them back together. Although this was probably frustrating for her at times, she was supportive. In adolescence this curiosity led to a fascination with computers and I began to build them and became quite good at fixing an array of problems ranging from household appliances to engines and computers. I think this foundation was a natural Segway into my interest in the human anatomy.

As a child growing up in Long Island, I always had a unique opportunity before me, something that most other people don't have these days. My father was the owner of a successful business that was given to him by his father.

My grandfather was a very dedicated man with enough business sense to start a business that would benefit later generations of the family. My grandfather was a Seabee in the Navy and they were considered the mechanics of the armed forces. During the 1940s as the country was recovering from the Great Depression and with World War II still very much on people's minds, my grandfather started his own marina. He worked incredibly long hours doing back breaking work. He knew that what he was building was something that would help his family for generations. My dad took over the business and it was always assumed that at some point, I would run the family marina. Both my dad and grandfather were very talented mechanics and self-taught engineers, which was the ideal environment for my own natural instincts in this area to flourish. With two sisters who never had an interest in the business, it was pretty much a given that I would become the owner and operator someday.

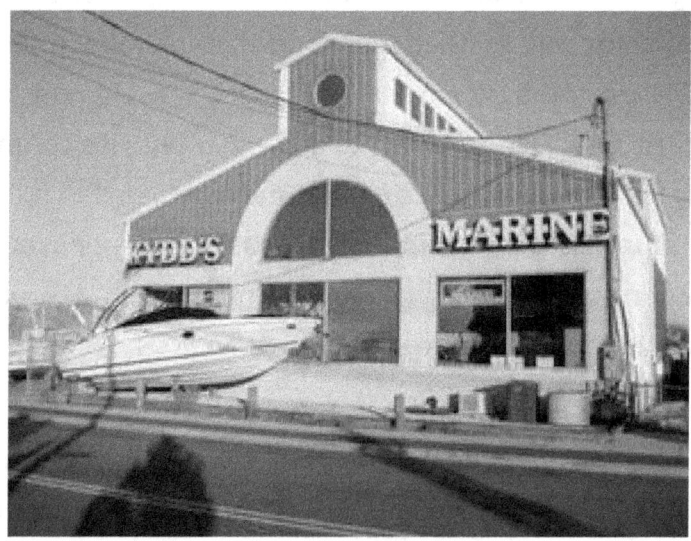

*Kydd's Marine, Massapequa NY*

When I was 8 or 9 years old, I began working at my family's marina doing manual labor. My primary work wasn't exactly stressful, but it was definitely work to a kid. I didn't have Tom Sawyer's ability to make work look desirable either – it never would have dawned on me that anyone else should do my work. My work was helping the family, and I didn't exactly mind the work or, at least, not all of it. Painting boats can be enjoyable, especially in the beginning. I was less enthusiastic about cleaning the boats because scraping the barnacles was hard work. Still, it was simply what was expected of me and I didn't question it.

Over the years I watched my father working more than 10 hours every day, seven days a week. He didn't take vacations and worked through a lot of holidays.

By comparison, I looked at my mother's family and began to notice just how much time they had to do what they wanted to do. They were white collar workers, primarily doctors and lawyers. I had an idea of what they did (or at least I thought I did). They were paid well, and they took their families on vacations and had stories about the holidays.

It was a very jarring observation for a child to make. I knew that I would take over the marina, but the idea of working long hours like my father really did not appeal to me. Living like my mother's side of the family did. I was just a kid though, so I really didn't think too much about it. Instead, I would get lost in my geeky little world when I wasn't at school or the marina. I played Dungeons & Dragons with my friends and read books. Deciding what I wanted to do was still so far away that I did not feel pressured to think much about it.

I grew up in a Catholic home, and we attended mass every Sunday. We weren't the most active family in the Church, there simply wasn't time. My mom had a personality that many people were always drawn to in the community and she was often a source of support not only in the church, but with her friends and even my friends as I grew older. When we did participate in Church activities, I found myself thoroughly enjoying how we helped others. I believe that watching my mom help people in this way inspired my desire to be of service.

When I reached high school, I started to look around my world again. Sure, I enjoyed my quiet activities with a close-knit group of friends. I was shy, and the idea of putting myself out there was terrifying. To say I was reserved would be an understatement. But I also felt like my life didn't have much in the way of direction. Sure, there was a blueprint that I could easily follow, letting my life just play itself out without me having to think or do too much about it. The teenage years are always quite the experience though. You start to question everything as the future gets so much closer.

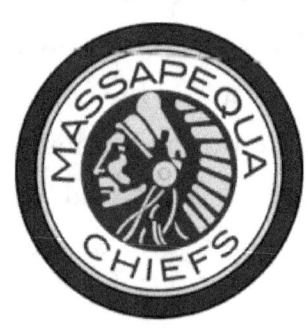

Acting in the usual teenage spirit of doing something new and different, I decided to join my high school football team. I wasn't big or in the best shape of my life, but I had potential. My sophomore year, I started playing football and quickly found an activity that I could really enjoy. It wasn't something someone told me to do, and it wasn't assumed that I should just do it. My parents were very supportive, letting me do what I wanted to do. They didn't make demands because they always wanted me and my sisters to be happy. If I wanted to play football, they were more than happy to support that. If nothing else, it was a great way to get me outside and exercising.

I loved it.

Playing football was like nothing else I had ever done. Almost every other member of the team had been playing football for years, so they already knew everything they needed to know. They were honing their skills as I began to absorb everything I could about the sport.

The biggest change for me was having a coach. It was not what I had expected, and it was certainly not like anything else I had ever experienced. For the first time in my life, there was someone who told me exactly what I needed to do to achieve a particular goal. He helped me overcome my reservations and start to talk with the team members – it's incredibly difficult to remain shy when you are on the field running at someone on the opposing team. I knew that I needed to have some kind of connection with my team to be effective, and the coach helped me get to a point where I was finally comfortable. We went to church before games and got up early to practice. There was a relatively strict schedule that drove my days instead of a vague idea of where I was headed. It was also an experience that made me far tougher than I had ever been before I attended high school. I loved all of it, especially the physical activity.

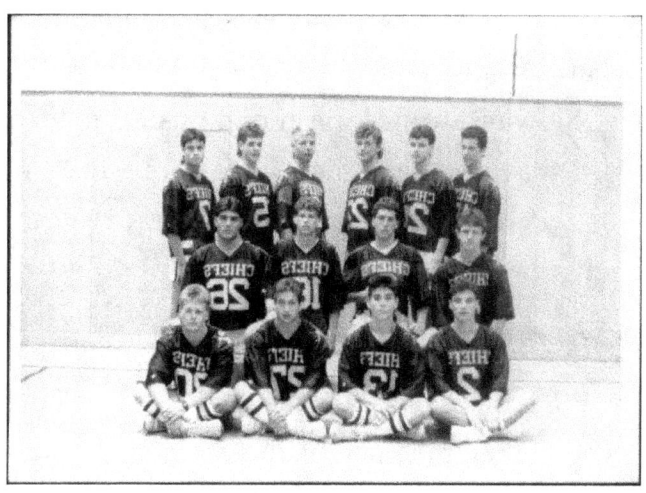

*Lacrosse team, 1988*

Only a few months after I started playing, we headed to the gym to work out for regular training. It was the standard activities, weights and cardio. I lay down to do some leg press exercises. As I brought the weights back down, there was a shooting pain in my neck. It was so bad that I stopped working out and went home.

When I told my mom about the pain and that I could not even turn my neck for the blinding pain, she immediately took me to the family doctor. It is a humbling experience as a teenager to find yourself suddenly unable to turn your head at all. That is the kind of thing that adults complain about. Yet there I was, on my way to our family doctor's office with an injury I sustained at the gym because of what I now know was improper positioning.

If I had thought that things couldn't get much worse, I would have been wrong. As it was, I was in so much pain I really wasn't thinking about much else. We went to my family doctor who practiced out of his home back then – it was common. He immediately said get to the ER, where they x-rayed and cat scanned my neck. After looking at the CAT scan and x-rays that the hospital had taken our doctor said that the top vertebrae in my neck was pinching a nerve, causing the excruciating pain. I was put in traction to take the pressure off of the nerve, and put on muscle relaxers and pain medication. For several weeks I just lay in the hospital room waiting for the pain to go away, or at least lessen. I was missing school, work, and football. When they finally decided to discharge me – with the pain every bit as severe as when I had gone into the hospital – they gave me a neck brace.

You can imagine what it was like for a teenager showing up to school with a neck brace.

The teasing was relentless. I had no comebacks because even I knew that I looked ridiculous. My best friend Omur enjoyed (and still does) making cartoons of me during this time period.

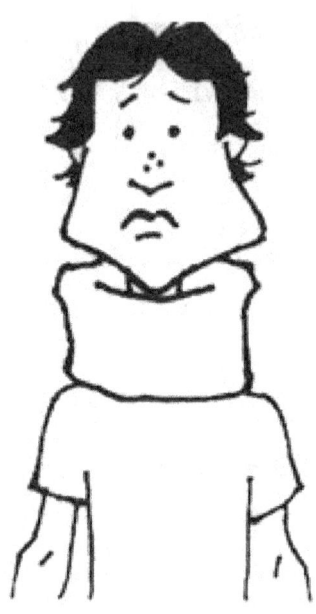

*Omur's Favorite Drawing*

Walking around with that massive contraption on my neck made it impossible for people not to notice me passing by in the hall or by a classroom door. Of course, I joined in the ribbing because what else could I do? I could fully appreciate how ridiculous the whole thing was. The only thing that bothered me was the fact that the pain was not getting better. The teasing was actually a nice distraction, and at least I wasn't still trapped in a hospital bed. A few months of playing football was more than long enough for me to get accustomed to regular exercise, so being trapped in a bed was like its own kind of torture. I much preferred walking around like a human giraffe, if only the pain would go away.

About a month after the injury, my dad decided that it was time to try something else. One of our family friends was a chiropractor who worked out of his home. He had even sponsored my dad for some boat races a few times. He had no problem loaning us the boat, and that was really the way I had viewed the doctor until that day.

We arrived at the doctor's home office. My dad explained what had happened, with some input and corrections from me, then explained the hospital's diagnosis and treatment. Of course, the doctor asked for the x-rays so that he could see for himself what was going on with my neck. That was pretty much all it took for him to know what to do. This was very different, so treatments were a little less ... gentle. He put me in something that is most easily described as the medical version of a headlock. The good doctor then realigned the vertebrae. It was like the most bizarre version of magic I had ever experienced, but the end results were exactly what I had hoped would happen at the hospital. The pain was significantly reduced. I could even turn my head again (with a bit of discomfort).

For $10, the doctor had done what weeks in a hospital and embarrassment at school had absolutely failed to achieve. I was finally on the road to recovery.

I returned for a few more session – no more than half a dozen – and by the end of it all, about 90% of the pain was gone. It would take another year or so for the pain to totally disappear, but I was again fully mobile. Little did I know how profoundly this experience would influence my future.

I continued to play football. I earned a mechanics license and started to do more important work at the marina. Things seemed to be going along in a much more satisfactory direction. For a few years, I was fairly happy with the way my life was shaping up, having learned just how bad things could be.

My college major at the time was business, which I had absolutely no interest in studying but thought it was a logical choice given the expectation of taking over the marina. Somewhere in the back of my mind, I still saw my mother's side of the family and was thinking that was the right direction to go in. The problem was that it wasn't really a direction. I was in college, but I wasn't doing particularly well, mostly because I didn't feel inspired by what I was studying. I felt a bit lost and something inside me knew that I was not on the right path. I was just going along without any real destination.

During spring break of my sophomore year, I was home visiting my family and working at the marina. Then a family friend arrived. Instead of the chiropractor who had fixed my neck about four years earlier, it was his son, who had become a doctor and taken over the practice. He was seeking to purchase a boat from his father. With time on his hands, he stopped to chat and we started talking about the future. He was a bit older than me and doing quite well for himself, making him a clear and independent voice; a new perspective for my dilemma about my future plans. I told him that I was in school, not doing particularly well and I was thinking about switching my major to become a physical therapist. He immediately waved away the idea, saying I would be much better off going for something a bit more specialized. As a chiropractor, his father helped a much wider group of people, but he could also do physical therapy if he wanted to practice that branch.

It was a light bulb moment in my life.

I told him that I remembered his father and how he had fixed my problem after weeks in the hospital had failed to help me. His words really struck a chord. For the next few months I thought about the idea of switching my major, doing a bit of research into what I would need to do (although he had provided some details to point me in the right direction). Before I started my junior year, I applied to a school in faraway Atlanta, Georgia, called Life University. Having lived all of my life in Long Island, if I were accepted it would be the first time that I would really be leaving home. When I submitted my application, I had no real thought as to what it would mean if I were accepted. I told no one of my decision to apply. Not my parents, not my sisters, and certainly not my girlfriend.

My girlfriend was visiting me when I received a call from the admissions office. I had been accepted and would be starting just after the New Year began. Understandably furious that I had not talked to her about my application, she did not have any words of congratulations for me. My parents were surprised, but, as always, incredibly supportive. With only four weeks before school was set to start, my mom helped me get everything together. I dropped out of the college I was attending on Long Island. With the car loaded up and ready to go, my mother and I began the long trip down the east coast to a completely different world.

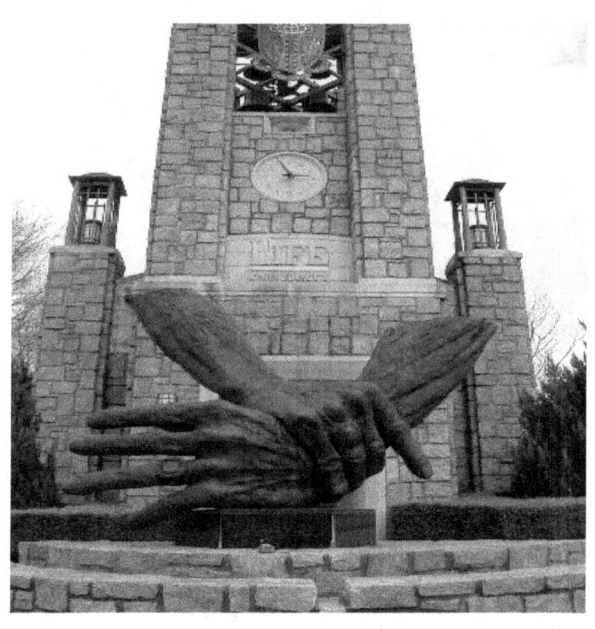

*Life University*

It probably comes as no surprise that my girlfriend broke up with me not too long thereafter.

There is no point when I have ever regretted the decision to go through with the change in schools. My focus for most of the next decade was on one thing – getting my degree. Just as I had learned to set goals with my coach in high school, I finally had another goal to work toward. I finally knew what I wanted to do, and I did not want to waste any time before making sure it became a reality. I felt inspired by the study of the human body. As I started to learn more, I finally felt I was on the right path to satisfy my natural curiosity about the inner workings of people. That same curiosity easily translated into the biomechanics of the human body.

My favorite place in school was the cadaver lab where I was able to dissect the human body and see how it worked. As I reflect on my early childhood, I now realize that the natural curiosity that was always there began to grow into my desired career. From the time I began taking classes at Life University until I earned my doctorate was 7.5 years. My degree was specific to the industry, a DC (Doctor of Chiropractic).

In June of 1996 at the age of 26, I opened the doors of my clinic.

What I had learned during that 7.5 years of higher education was more than enough to give me the skills and knowledge to help people. However, I have always had the desire to know and learn more, so I spent many hours doing post graduate work at specialty seminars and workshops. I was again getting a sense of satisfaction from my job. This time it was because of something I chose to do. Having been through my own painful injury, I knew just how my patients felt, or at least how most of them felt. The pain that had seemed destined to follow them for the rest of their lives had a solution.

I was content, and business was good.

Then I suffered a debilitating and humbling injury that traditional chiropractic methods were not able to help me with. I was helping move 50-pound sandbags when I was reminded that I was not as young as I once was. As a result of moving about 1,200 pounds of sand, I had herniated a disc in my lower back (between L4 and L5). Lower back pain is *the* leading cause of injuries that result in missing work. I knew that. Yet it did not stop it from happening to me. For two days I could not move, not even to get up to go to the bathroom. Again confined to my bed, it was like being tortured all over again. I had to have my office closed because I could not do anything for my patients. Unlike the last time though, I had a fairly good idea of what was wrong and who I should call. I had a number of friends in my field, so I called one of them (after I had unsuccessfully tried another chiropractor). He was conducting research into lower back pain, which made him an ideal chiropractor to help me resolve the problem. . My friend, Dave, showed up, and just like with my father's friend, he was able to fix things in less than an hour. It took a little longer than my first experience (about 30 minutes), but it was more than just my neck this time. Even though I had been bedridden for a couple of days, he managed to have me up and walking shortly after he arrived. This experience inspired another career change that would lead me to widen my scope of practice. The unexpected career change would allow me to help people in a way that chiropractic methods alone could not.

This time I did not sit on what I had learned from my experience. There was no question about what I wanted to do. The methods that Dave used and my immediate relief of symptoms inspired me to learn more so that I could have even more tools at my disposal. Dave's work included injections. This experience opened my eye to the emerging field of medicine called regenerative medicine. I earned another degree in Acupuncture, earned a nursing license, and finally a degree as a nurse practitioner. All of this was necessary, though not unpleasant. For example, to become a registered nurse (RN), I went to school in Florida for a year. My family remained in Arizona and my business continued to operate as usual while I pursued my studies. Most of my time was dedicated to the extremely exacting and demanding work required to become an RN, but at least the environment was different, even pleasant when it wasn't hurricane season. I began working on my master's degree. This was what I had been working for – the ability to administer regenerative medicine and PRP, stem cells injections. This is what had fixed my problems, and I wanted to pass on my experience to others. Twice traditional means had failed me, resulting in a lot of lost time and work. As well as a healthy helping of embarrassment in both cases (it isn't much better to be a chiropractor out with a hurt back as it is to be a student with a neck brace).

I have been through the pain that others have experienced, and in both cases, it taught me just what the right treatment can do. Everyone is different, and the same solution is not going to work for everyone. Even worse, when we get complacent, we fail to make progress. Accepting that things are working just fine is never a justification to always follow tradition. To the old adage "If it isn't broke don't fix it," I say it might be broke and you just don't realize it until you have to experience it. With as resilient as the human body is, there is always a better solution, you just have to find it.

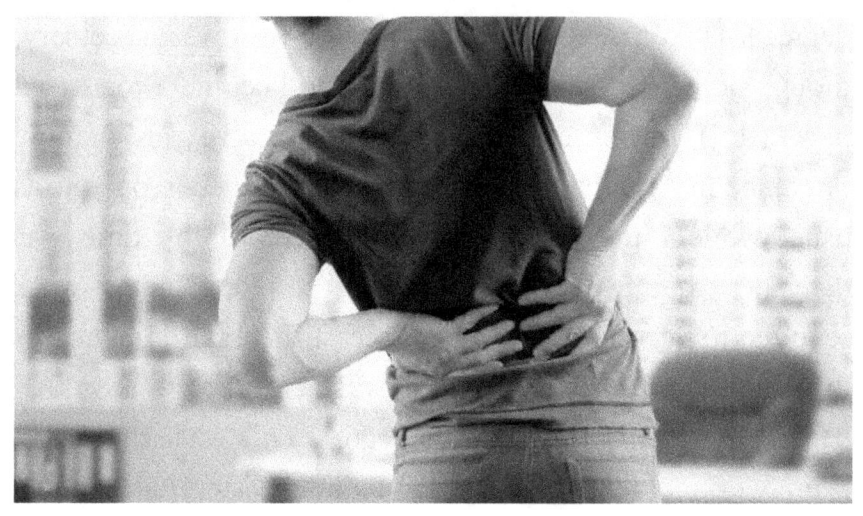

*Back Pain can be disabling*

The expectation in technology is that it will always go forward, that we will always need something new to replace what is working just fine now. And that is acceptable. There is no reason to feel any differently about the medical profession. When it comes to pain and the current medical model of treatment I don't see it moving forward. I see many failed back surgeries, opioid addiction, and outdated insurance driven procedures. During the Victorian Era, they would literally bleed patients to treat them, and they believed that it worked just fine. When it comes to the human body, there are far more reasons to question what is currently accepted when it keeps us from moving forward.

We have reached a time when the accepted solution is almost always to medicate problems instead finding the cause and treating it. Medication is acceptable up to a point to help ease pain – it absolutely is not meant to be the final solution though. The end result of this kind of thinking has given rise to one of the worse epidemics of our time: the opioid epidemic. Since pain killers simply mask the pain, there is no known end to the length of time the drugs will be needed by patients.

Although effective, even my old method of treatment could not help everyone, which I learned in part due to my own injury. I understood that the problem needed to be treated, and I began to question the best way to do that. I had learned a small part of the treatment spectrum (granted it was all of the available knowledge when I was at the university), and I did not see a need to entirely rethink my approach until I had a harsh reminder of why you should always look at your profession from a different perspective. I have always done a lot of continuing education, but without a medical degree I could not practice regenerative medicine. It took going through an injury and pain again to realize how much more I could be doing for my patients. Sure, I was helping many of them feel better. Still, there was more I could do.

Just like my 15-year-old self who stepped into my family friend's office, patients who arrive at my door have already been through so much. Doctors and hospitals have used various traditional methods, putting the patients through the wringer. The focus is almost always on pain management instead of healing the body. After being reminded of the reason why it was important to keep learning, I finally have a way to treat patients that will not require them to return to my office regularly for the rest of their lives.

The methods that I have learned from my additional years in school have included some very effective treatments that are not invasive and are proving to be very successful at helping people recover from their injuries. The injections that I use to treat patients in pain are regenerative, helping the body to heal instead of masking the pain. I have already been down that road. I lay in bed for weeks as a teenager, uncomfortable and restless, while my body was expected to "right" itself. When it didn't, a neck brace was supposed to encourage my body to heal on its own. Pain does not work that way. You should not ignore it or mask it, hoping that the root cause will miraculously heal. As often as not, it will heal incorrectly, if at all. There are few things that I have done that have been more rewarding than working with a patient who has been through severe pain and surgery (or surgeries) and seeing that patient finally experience a better quality of life. Patients don't need heavy medication because their bodies are finally starting to repair themselves.

To break the cycle of pain, you have to fix the root cause. It is a science that will likely always be moved forward. To me, that solution today is through the use of regenerative methods, including physical rehabilitation, chiropractic, acupuncture, and regenerative injections. It is a natural, non-addictive approach. I have seen the changes in the lives of people who have suffered severe or crippling pain for years. My extensive training in traditional, holistic, and regenerative medicine have given me the unique ability to diagnose and apply a multi-therapeutic approach to complicated pain patients. Offering this kind of broader scope of treatment to those who are suffering is the future of treating pain, and it is evolving faster than I am able to write about it. Instead of masking, medicating, and removing diseased and damaged tissues, the new and more efficient treatments are evolving into regenerating and rehabilitating damaged and diseased tissues.

My intent with this book is to provide a resource of all of your options to help you understand the full range so that you can make a more informed decision on what is right for you. This is a more complete look at the new methods and more traditional treatments that actually treat the problem.

# CHAPTER 2

# A Bit of Anatomy: Understanding the Back and Why It Is So Easy to Injure?

Most of us take our backs for granted, and while we are young that seems to be just fine. There will be a price, but that is so far down the road that you shouldn't be concerned, right? If you are no longer considered young, you already know the answer – the price is far too steep and never at quite the old age you expect.

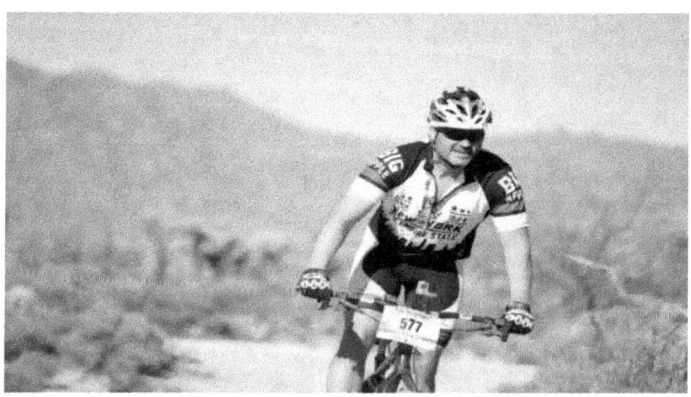

*It's the Little Things*

So why is it that we seem to go along with doing everything without any problems, then suddenly our backs decide that they simply cannot continue as they always have, making it difficult to do even the most mundane tasks? I've known someone who was in fairly good shape and in his 40s, and it appeared that all things were fine. Then one day he was in real pain and was hesitant to tell me exactly what happened, saying that it was too embarrassing. When he finally did spit the reason out, I could understand why he felt that he should keep it to himself. He had managed to strain a muscle in his back by simply putting on his pants earlier in the week.

It's something that they don't tell you when you are young. As you age, if you have not properly taken care of your back, you can put too much pressure on a nerve or pinch a nerve in your back in the most embarrassing and seemingly mundane ways possible.

Even worse than feeling embarrassed, you will be in a lot of pain and will not be able to do other tasks (even ordinary ones) without causing yourself further pain. Whether or not it is too late, there are things you can do to stabilize your back so that you don't have the same problems later. Chapter 9 goes into detail about what you can do, but for the most part these are things that you already know you *should* be doing:

- Sit up straight
- Stand up and move around at least once an hour
- Don't cross your legs
- Get regular exercise

There is a lot more to it, but those are the basics if you want to get started now without having to read all of Chapter

9 first. The chapter provides details on what good posture is, the kinds of exercises to do (both if your back is fine and additional exercises for those who are experiencing back pain), and other behaviors that will strengthen your core and hips to better support your back.

Don't worry, I'm not going to be discussing a lot of details about the anatomy of the back. You will get just enough information to help you understand the injuries and types of treatments typically recommended. With three very different aspects working together to let you accomplish everything you do, you do need to know at least the basics. Whether you suffer from lower back problems, a pinched nerve, tension headaches or an old injury, understanding how these three components work together (or in some cases against each other) will give you a better understanding of what you can do to provide better support for your back. This will go a long way to help you treat the root problem instead of simply coping with the pain. Most of the time, people can significantly reduce the pain by simply being more aware of how they are hurting their backs.

# The Spine – An Overview

The human spine has a lot of different components and is an essential part in nearly every movement you make. From sitting and sleeping to exercising and moving, your back is instrumental in everything you do. Each of the components of the back are involved in all of your activities. There are three primary aspects of the spine, any of which can be the source of pain that you feel as you age:

- The muscles
- Thejoints
- The nerves

Each of these is instrumental in everything you do every day. All three components work together to keep you moving, and all three of them can cause debilitating pain. You can easily avoid a lot of the pain associated with each of these parts of the back by taking care of your back.

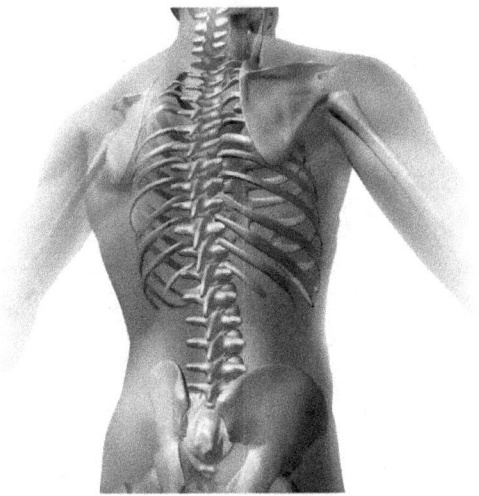

*The Spine*

## The Muscles

The muscles are easily the largest aspect of the back (besides your skin), your back muscles are often where you are going to feel the pain when things start to hurt. Many muscles of the back are actually part of your appendages. This is why you can easily hurt your back with the wrong kinds of moves, too.

The following are the major muscles of the back:

- The trapezius is named after the shape of the muscle, and you have two: one on each side of your spine. It starts with the neck around the base of the skull down the shoulder and about half way down your spine.
- The teres major stretches from the shoulder blade to the shoulder. The muscle helps you rotate the humerus (your upper arm).
- The teres minor is one of the muscles of the rotator cuff. When you raise your arm, this muscle flexes.
- Latissimus dorsi covers much of the lower back, and has a little overlap with the trapezius.
- Levator scapulae is like a strap that stretches down the neck to the scapula.
- Rhomboid major and minor run parallel to each other (F is rhomboid major). These muscles stretch from the spine to the shoulder blade.

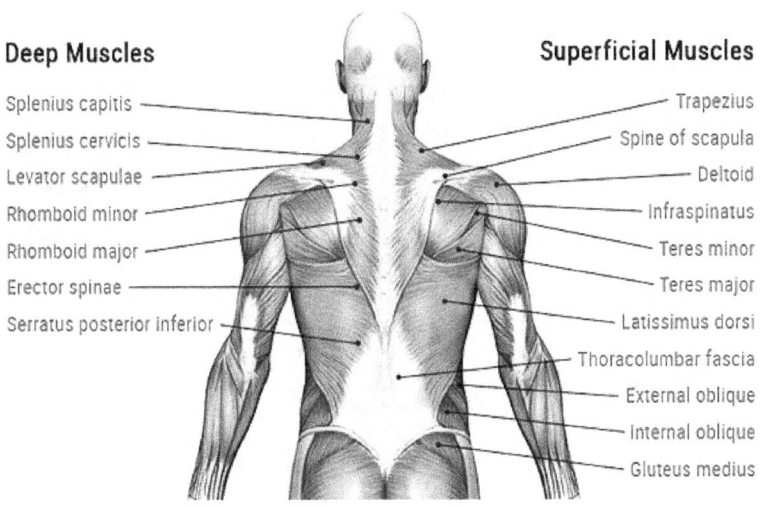

*The Main Back Muscles*

Your spine acts as a mirror, with each of these major muscles appearing in the same place on either side of your spine. Considering how much these muscles do every day, this is a fairly small number of muscles.

Often the most common pains are related to a person straining or spraining one or several of these muscles. Lower back pain and tension headaches are frequently caused by over use of the affected muscles, improper lifting or motions, or lack of motion, all of which can hurt your muscles. Lack of exercise is one of the leading causes of muscle strain and sprain. Muscle pains are usually accompanied by spasms, which can be distracting even when the pain is dull.

# The Spine

The spine, often called the backbone and vertebral column, is a long series of bones that is divided into five main sections, and runs from the spine to the bottom of the torso. This long, essential part of your body includes 24 vertebrae. Between each of the vertebra are intervertebral discs that absorb the shock that your body experiences all day, acting as a shock absorber as you go about your daily activities.

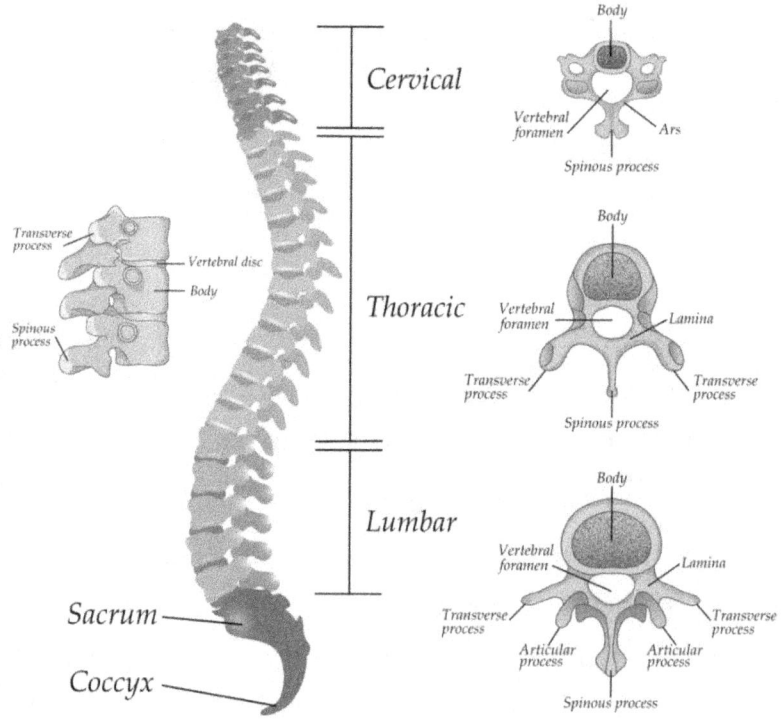

*The Complexity of the Spine*

The different sections of the spine have slightly different types of vertebrae:

- The cervical section of the spine is the top area, or the part of the spine in your neck.

- The thoracic is the largest section and your ribs are attached to this part of your spine.

- The lumbar is the portion of the spine between the ribs and pelvis. You've probably heard of the lumbar section of the back because it is the part that most people hurt while they are doing mundane tasks. If you experieince lower back pain, there are good odds that these vertabrae are affected, if not part of the cause. Unlike the thoracic and sacrum, there aren't other supporting bone structures, meaning that your lumbar has to work much harder to support you. This is why you want to have strong stomach muscles. They can offer the kind of support your lumbar needs to keep from unnecessary wear and tear.

- The sacrum connects to the hip bones and is fully fused, making it more difficult to hurt than the upper areas of the spine.

- The coccyx is usually called the tail bone. The vertebrae are fused here, but it is more succeptible to harm since you can hurt it by falling on it. This can be incredibly painful, although it is not very common.

While muscles primarily help you to move different parts of your body, your spine fulfills four primary functions:

- The spine is what supports everything above your hips. It carries the weight of your entire upper body, and anything that you are carrying.

- It works as the central axis for your body

- All movement that includes turning your head or your torso is possible because of your spine. Any sedentary activities you do are also managed by your spine, and it is the hours of sitting that can be the most punishing for this part of your body.

- The bones of the spine are also what protect all of the nerves of the spinal cord. When the vertebrae of the spine sit on the nerves (commonly referred to as a pinched nerve), it causes severe, often excruciating pain. This was what happened to me during my first season playing football in high school.

When your back hurts, the vast majority of the time it will be as a result of some issue with your spine. Even muscle spasms can be alleviated by realigning the spine. This is the reason why people visit chiropractors for back pain; most of the pain can be alleviated in the short-term by realigning the bones.

## The Nerves

Running along most of the length of your spine are a bundle of nerves, tissues, and cells that branch out into every other part of your body. In the worst cases, damage to your spine can cause paralysis because the injury can permanently damage the nerves in your spine. The spinal cord is the second part of the central nervous system (the first part is your brain). Everything that you think you want to do is accomplished by your decision being sent from your brain down the spinal cord to whatever body part you want to move. Even as I sit here typing this paragraph, my brain and spinal cord are hard at work telling my fingers what to do, and which keys to press as my eyes read each of the words. It's absolutely fascinating how many things your brain does at the same time. It is just as impressive when you consider how your spinal cord helps you to do things like play sports, hike take pictures, and swim. All of these activities are possible because of that bundle of nerves hidden in the bones of your spine.

This is why pinched nerves can be so disabling, keeping you from being able to move your head, legs, or arms. When the vertebrae are out of alignment or a disc is herniated, it can keep the messages from your brain from reaching the intended area.

This does not mean that you should ignore pain or try to power through the pain though. The longer you ignore pain, the more likely it is you will experience longer-lasting damage.

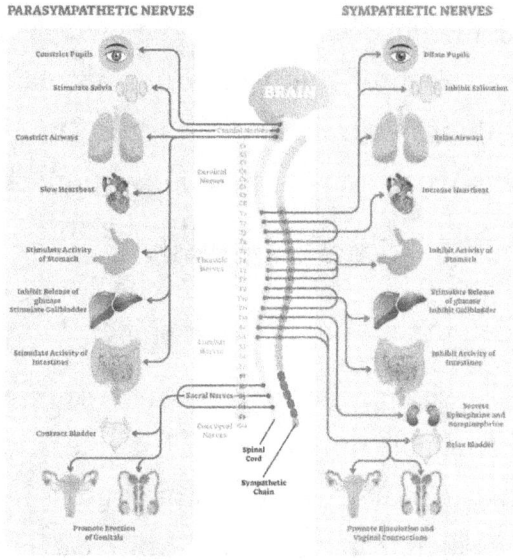

*The Spinal Cord connects all organs*

There are many different aspects and a lot of technical jargon that go with the spinal cord – it is a major part of your body. However, it is not necessary to know about these terms to understand back pain. It is enough to know that most of the nerves in your body lead back to the spinal cord, which is protected by the bones of your spine. Back pain that involves the nerves is almost always caused by a problem with the spine and its surrounding structures, which restrict or push on the nerves, causing the severe to debilitating pain that will certainly force you to go to a doctor or the hospital.

# Why Backs Are So Easy to Injury

Backs are incredibly easy to hurt *because* we take them for granted. Pretty much everything we do requires some work for our backs. Even sleeping requires our spines and muscles to work. The more time we spend sitting in office chairs and being sedentary, the more stress and strain we put on our backs. When we decide we don't have time to exercise, it is our backs that will pay for this (as well as most of the rest of our bodies, but somewhat ironically most people don't correlate lack of exercise with hurting the back). We seem to think that the less active we are, the easier we make it for our backs, which simply isn't true.

Consider how your legs feel after sitting in the car for hours. They are stiff and may protest when you try to stand up – and this only gets worse as you get older. When you sit at a desk, you are much more likely to shift positions, move your legs, and do other activities that will keep them from getting too stiff. Most of us do not do this for our backs.

An initial study has found that people in developing countries who do manual labor are less likely to suffer from the regular pain and discomfort of white collar workers in developed nations who sit in ergonomic chairs for hours every day. Part of this is that the people who do manual labor stay active, which keeps their muscles more toned and does not put the same stress on their backs for about eight hours a day. They change positions, are more likely to stretch, and generally are more aware of any pain from the beginning.

If you are very active over the weekend after being sedentary all week, you are really setting yourself up for pain later. You have to work out every day instead of relying on two days of intense physical labor or working out.

Over time, your back simply isn't going to be able to take all of the stress and pressure of sitting. It will start to show signs of the long-term damage through dull aches, then it will progress to tweaked nerves and muscle spasms. You should take all pain seriously, especially when it is in your back. If you won't listen to the experts about exercising and sitting properly, you should listen to your own body. It is really quite easy to prevent the kind of pain that most people suffer by simply acting in a way that is more natural for humans. We weren't designed for sitting for long periods of time, and your back is going to let you know that as you get older.

Do yourself a favor and be more careful about your daily activities. Sure, it is going to be annoying, even uncomfortable at first. Sitting up straight and maintaining good posture takes re-programming how you act. Not staring at your cell phone is going to be annoying. But in the long run, re-training yourself will literally save you a lot of pain later. All of the little things that you do incorrectly now are going to add up to pain that is much more serious later. And you have the ability to almost completely avoid back problems by properly taking care of your back.

Even if you are already suffering back pain, there are things you can do to start reducing that pain. Chapter 9 goes into this in more detail but, for now, you should start thinking about what it is that you do that is causing you pain. If you notice a little twitch of pain when you are putting on socks, that lets you know that you are moving in a way that is hurting your back, and you should consider it an omen of more pain to come if you don't start changing your habits.

There are three large components working together to keep you moving every day. If there is a problem with any one of these components, it can cause you a lot of discomfort or pain. When you get injured or have ignored the warning signs, the pain can become debilitating. It doesn't have to be as long as you start supporting your back as much as it supports you.

# CHAPTER 3

# Mechanics of Back Injury, Different Pain Drivers of Low Back Pain

Your back can sustain so many different types of injuries that it is nearly impossible to list them all. There are even more *ways* for you to injure your back, including while you are just doing some of the most mundane activities. Ultimately though, back pain is rarely something that happens suddenly – most pain is the result of months (or more often years) of wear and tear on your back. There are definitely some types of pain that you cannot avoid, but you can minimize the pain.

For now, let's just focus on the types of injuries and the resulting pain from them. Most people are well aware that there are different kinds of pain – a dull headache is nothing compared to the immediate pain you feel after stubbing your toe. When it comes to your back, it is very important that you are able to explain to your doctor about the type of pain that you are experiencing. Any history of injuries to your back that you have had is also going to be critical to helping determine the source of the pain and anything that contributes to it.

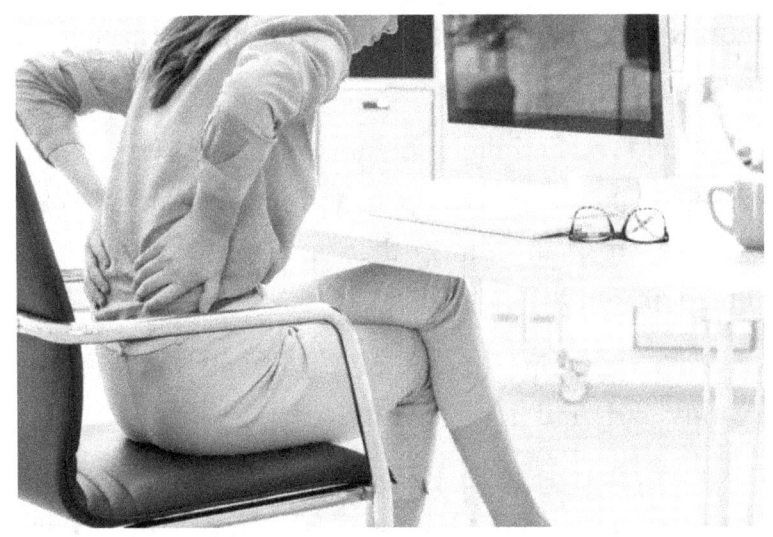

*Your Back Is One of Your Biggest Assets – Take Care of It*

# Different Types of Pain

The thing about pain is that it comes in so many different types and intensities. For most people, back pain has a slow start that builds over time. Then there is the more sudden and debilitating types of pain that you cannot ignore, that interrupts everything until you are successfully treated. It's an enormous range that encompasses every kind of pain imaginable, which clearly makes it more difficult to figure out exactly what is wrong. That's one reason why any kind of back pain should lead you to seek help from a medical professional.

### Your Body and Pain

Before diving into the types of back pain you may experience, let's take a quick look at the three primary categories of pain. These types of pain apply to your entire body, not just to your back.

While you definitely should seek professional help, you should also understand your pain and injuries because in most cases there are many things that you can do that will help minimize or remove the pain.

There are three types of pain (and this is true for everybody part, and not just your back).

- Nociceptive pain affects tissues and usually comes from an outside source, such as a bee sting or illness. Conditions like arthritis are also considered a kind of nociceptive pain. Any pain that you feel when you change your position or adjust the load on a particular body part is nociceptive. Usually, the pain is dull or it reduces significantly after the initial injury.

- Neuropathic pain directly affects the nervous system. From something as common as striking your funny bone (which has a very different feeling to hitting your shin on a coffee table) to multiple sclerosis to the side effects of alcoholism, there are a lot of potential sources for this kind of pain. The focus is on what part of your body is affected. This kind of pain tends to be residual and often never fully heals because nerves don't really heal like the rest of your body does.

- Other types of pain will probably be the easiest to remember because they don't have a scientific name. This kind of pain comes from neurological dysfunction that may or may not affect a person's neurological system. These are the kinds of ailments that have often been ignored by the medical profession for decades or even centuries before finally being recognized. Diseases like fibromyalgia, complex regional pain syndrome, and irritable bowel syndrome fall into this category. The pains in this category are usually mild or re-occurring. For most of medical history, these kinds of ailments were considered to be normal aging ailments, but recently they have gained attention because there really isn't anything normal about constant pain. As stated earlier, all pain is a sign that something is wrong and should not be ignored. For now, names are being applied to the various types of pain as the medical profession finally starts trying to determine the causes for the many residual, low-grade pain ailments.

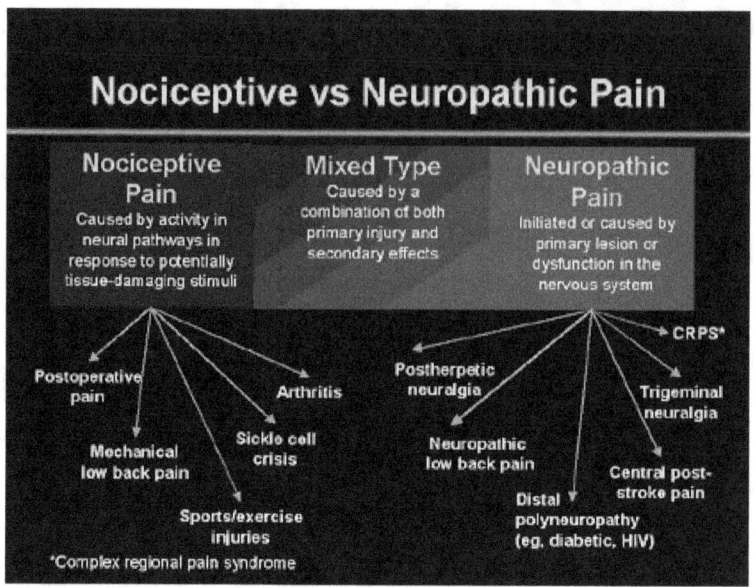

*The Three Types of Pain*

It's important to understand these three types of pain because some of the pain you experience in your other body parts may originate from your back. Obviously, if you suffer from Irritable Bowel Syndrome, that is not related to a problem with your back. If you have fibromyalgia though, you may dismiss a pain in your leg because the ailment does not have any kind of predictability. However, if the pain is different than what you are accustomed to, it may be a problem with your back, and not fibromyalgia. It is possible that fibromyalgia could exacerbate the problem, but if you have a shooting pain in your leg or foot, it could be related to a problem with your spine, such as a pinched nerve.

There are many kinds of ways to classify pain because there are so many different ways to experience the way you are hurting. We could discuss quick and slow pains (an injury versus soreness) or visceral (organ) and somatic (bones, joints, muscle, and skin), but for this book these three classifications are more than adequate to help you understand your back pain. Any one of these three types of pain is recognizable as being a problem and should result in you heading to see your physician. This book simply gives you the ability to provide a little more detail about the pain you feel. Just like it is frustrating to communicate with a child who simply points to the pain and says "Ouch," it can be challenging for a doctor to figure out what is wrong when all you can say is that something hurts. No, you don't have to try to use the technical terms (when you are hurting, you probably won't remember the scientific terms anyway), but if you think you know the source of your pain or can better define the type of pain you are experiencing, that can help your doctor to eliminate a lot of potential problems and focus on the most likely scenarios.

## Understanding Your Back Pain

You can certainly experience all three types of pain in any body part. Over the course of your life, you are very likely to experience all three types of pain in your back (hopefully not at the same time). When it comes to the lower back, there is another set of designations you should know.

One of the most important things to know about back pain is that there is no such thing as a pain that doesn't have a cause. If you have a doctor who tells you that you have a degenerative disorder, you should translate that into your doctor has no idea what is wrong. Yes, every part of your body will function less optimally over time, but that is not a disease, that is simply wear and tear. If you are hurting, there is a reason, and your doctor needs to figure out what the actual problem is. In most cases, you will get better over time, as long as you find out what triggers the pain and learn how to counter it.

MRIs and x-rays can only do so much. For the majority of the different causes of back pain, the best way to identify the source is for the doctor to spend time with you trying to cause the pain. If the idea of intentionally making the pain flare up is a bit unsettling, then make sure to pay close attention to what you do that causes the pain. When you brush your teeth, notice if there is a twinge of pain as you lean forward. When you get dressed in the morning, notice how your back reacts to each movement you make to put on each article of clothing. There are a lot of components to putting on your clothes, making this a great time to understand the pain and what actions you make that trigger the pain.

Sometimes back pain gets so bad that you completely change how you walk to keep your back or neck from hurting. If it has gotten this bad, you have definitely waited too long and should seek medical help immediately. Changing how you walk means that you are redistributing the load to another part of your body, and over time this is going to cause you even more pain.

Once you reach your physician, you should prepare to experience the pain – this is necessary for your doctor to be able to figure out how to treat you. If your physician doesn't work to isolate the pain, you should probably look for a specialist who can determine the cause. The best place to start is to figure out where the stress is. Everyone is different, and what starts the pain in your back is specific to you. The exercises that you should do to deal with the pain are specific to what your triggers are. A full assessment will probably take far too long (the most thorough exam requires 3 hours), but there are a few things that a physician can have you do to determine what sets off the pain and what area is the most stressed by that trigger.

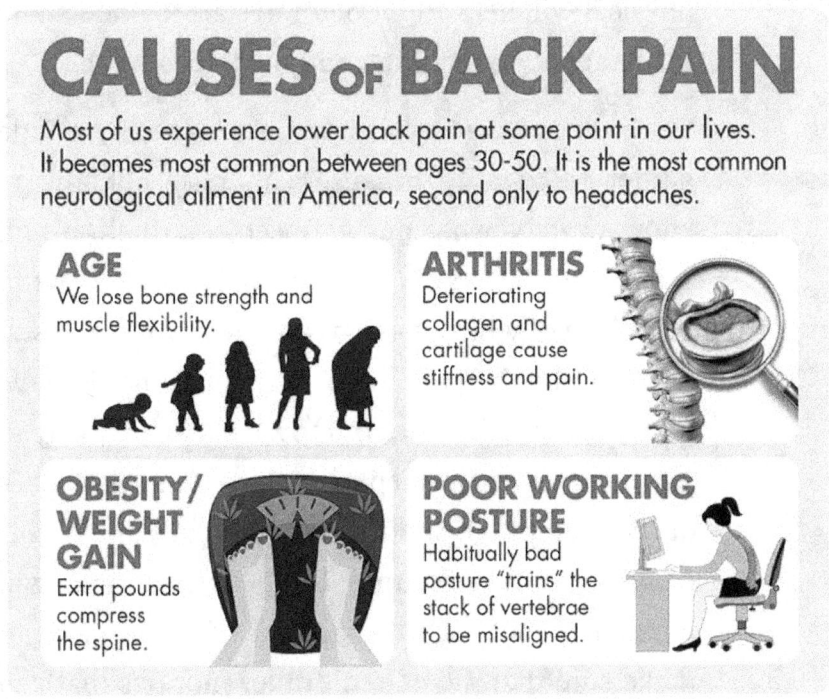

*Back Pain Is Specific to You and Your Habits*

What the medical professionals are going to look at is the motions that cause you the most pain, which postures enhance the pain, and loads that increase that pain. Sometimes the most telling thing will be the changes in movement that you have become accustomed to doing to avoid the pain.

- Your posture is not always a choice. Some athletes tend to keep their heads turned down, not because they are looking at their phones, but because there is a pain in their spine that they can alleviate through this posture. It isn't a great solution, and it can certainly cause other problems – this is where a physical will help your doctor to start to understand the pain and to recommend how to deal with it.

- The motions that result in pain are usually a little harder to identify because you may not always know exactly what angle, speed, or rotation will cause the pain. Still, you probably have a pretty good idea of which motions are most likely to result in triggering the pain. Your physician should have you go through a series of motions that are likely to set off pain, so be prepared. If you can provide a quick example of what is likely to cause pain, this could speed things up a bit. However, you will probably need to go through all of the motions to make sure that there aren't other motions that can also cause you pain.

- Your back is constantly managing different loads that you put on it over the course of the day. Load refers to the weight and force that you put on your back. Your vertebrae have a different reaction if they are injured, the muscles have a different reaction around injured areas, and shifting your weight can definitely exacerbate pain.

There are many factors that a physician needs to take into account when determining what the primary problem is with your back. The simple fact that you are aging is not the reason that your back hurts – there actually is a source, a reason for your pain. To address and treat it, you have to learn what you are doing that triggers it. From there, you will be able to build a healthier way to manage and treat the pain. Over time, the area of pain will gristle and strengthen so that it does not hurt anymore. That is why it isn't degenerative. It is also why you have to learn what the source of the problem is. To help your back to heal, you have to know how to strengthen your back without doing more harm.

Everyone is different, and your pain is not like anyone else's. Sure it can be classified, but the cause is unique to you and your lifestyle.

## When It Isn't Mechanical

Perhaps the most important reason to go through the pain is to understand the source of that pain. All back pain is sourced in an injury, a motion, a position, or a load. If you go through an assessment and you are not able to stimulate more pain or make it feel better, then the problem may not be with your back – it may not be a mechanical problem. Often an inability to stimulate and lessen pain during these assessments is a sign that you have something else wrong, such as a tumor or infection. They are not related to the mechanical workings of your back and cannot be triggered by movements, loads, or postures, and will require a completely different type of treatment to stop the pain.

## MECHANICAL BACK PAIN

- **Muscle, ligament, tendon strain**
- Discogenic disorders including herniated disc
- Apophyseal joint arthritis
- Spinal stenosis
- Spondylolysis, spondylolisthesis
- Scoliosis

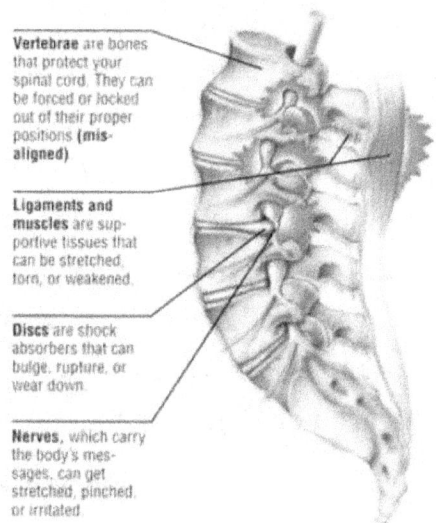

**Vertebrae** are bones that protect your spinal cord. They can be forced or locked out of their proper positions (misaligned)

**Ligaments and muscles** are supportive tissues that can be stretched, torn, or weakened.

**Discs** are shock absorbers that can bulge, rupture, or wear down.

**Nerves**, which carry the body's messages, can get stretched, pinched, or irritated.

*Not All Pain Is Mechanical in Nature*

# Risk Factors

Pretty much everything you do has associated risks for your back, but there are a lot of things that you probably do that exacerbate the problem or problems you will have later in life. You've been hearing people tell you to sit up straight and lift heavy objects properly all of your life, but the odds are that you don't follow what you know is meant to make things easier for your back. All of the things that you neglect to do are actually risks you are choosing to take because it is inconvenient to change the way you do things. This is going to be one of the hardest risks to mitigate because it requires not only reprogramming your behavior, but rethinking all of your regular activities to take your back into account.

I didn't say it would be easy, but if you do this while you are still young, you can forego the vast majority of pain that most people experience during their lives. When you consider the fact that back pain is the leading cause of people calling out sick to work, it is worth taking the time to rethink and reprogram your behavior. Prevention is definitely the best way to deal with back pain.

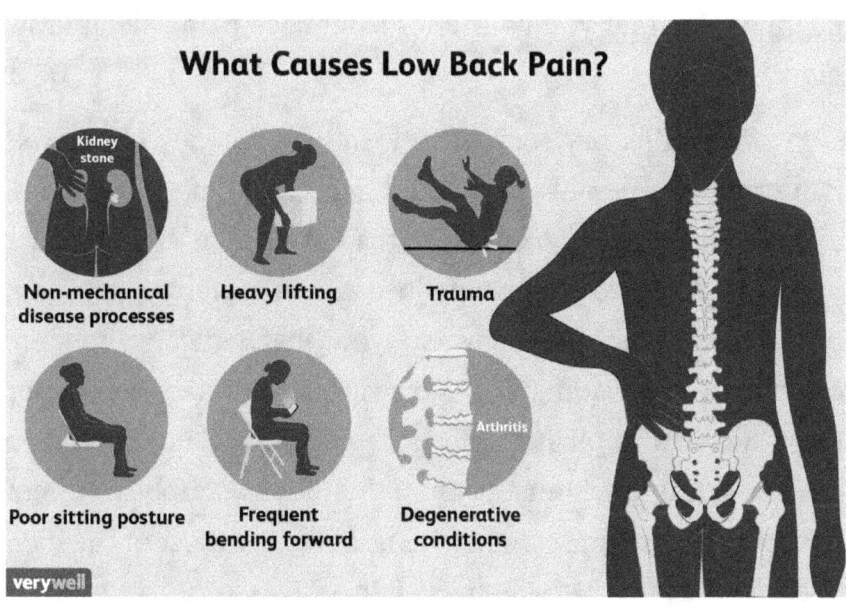

*All the Ways to Increase Wear and Tear on Your Back*

Beyond the behaviors that you already know you should be doing to reduce potential damage to your back, there are several other risks. These are risks that you already know address other aspects of your health. What you may not know is that they are things that can also be significant contributors to back pain, particularly pain of the lower back.

Exercise and diet – you knew this was coming – are clear contributors to back pain if they aren't taken seriously. If you are overweight, the additional weight is going to hurt your whole body, including your back. For people whose excess weight tends to go to their stomachs, you have even more motivation to take your caloric intake more seriously. The additional weight in the front directly affects your lower back, guaranteeing that you will suffer from back pain as you grow older.

Your diet plays a huge role in this, but lack of exercise is just as detrimental. You could actually argue that lack of exercise affects your back more than your diet. Not only are you more likely to gain weight because you aren't exercising, but the lack of movement on your back means you are essentially overloading it. Regular movement may work your back, but that is far healthier for your back than for you to remain sitting for hours at a time. Humans simply were not designed to remain seated or lying down for most of the day. We have always been active; with only a century or so of humans increasing the amount of time when they are idle, so your body is still not designed for it. There are many good reasons why you need to make sure you stand up at least once an hour. Even more importantly, you need to be taking a few walks each day for at least 15 minutes at a time. Your back needs that time to stretch and distribute the weight of your body differently. Naturally, your hips and legs also benefit from exercise because they need to move more often than they do when you are at a desk all day. We'll go into the ways to increase exercise and make sure you aren't over stressing your back by sitting for prolonged periods later in the book. For now, you should build frequent walks into your day. You need at least 30 minutes of solid exercise, but over the course of a work day, get up and walk around at least a few times. This does not count toward your daily exercise, but it does give you a break and helps you stretch. This also gives you a bit of time to clear your mind.

Those last two causes of back pain aren't exactly lesser known risks, so here is something you probably don't associate with back pain – smoking. If you are a smoker, you are hurting nearly every part of your body, including your back. Yes, your respiratory system is harmed the most, but smoking also reduces your blood flow. When you consider that the blood flow to your entire lower body has to travel through your lower back, it is easy to start to see how smoking can cause serious problems to your back. As your blood flow is reduced, fewer nutrients are delivered to the discs of your spine. This not only harms your back, but it reduces the healing process. It both helps create a problem and blocks the recovery.

Any disease you have could actively harm your back as well. The most obvious are ailments like scoliosis, which presents itself in the back, and arthritis that can affect your spine. Typically arthritis in the back begins with an injury, then the arthritis develops around the site of the injury, worsening over time. Cancer can also cause back pain, and as I have already mentioned, it can be far more difficult to detect and treat. It does not conform to the other kinds of back pain, and is not necessarily triggered by any particular action, movement, or position.

Another lesser known issue associated with back pain are psychological issues specifically anxiety and depression and trauma. What we understand about the relationship between the mind and body is still in its infancy, so exactly how these psychological conditions can cause or intensify pain is not known. There are many potential contributing factors, such as posture and excess tension, and you are less likely to exercise when you aren't feeling well mentally. Your body is definitely affected by your mental state, and pain is just one more manifestation of certain mental disorders. Major changes in your life, particularly those that are unexpected, can affect even the happiest person. When you are going through a difficult time, it could be well worth while to talk to a professional to ensure that you not only treat your mental anguish, but ensure that it doesn't spread to do you physical harm. My wife happens to be a therapist at world renowned treatment center for trauma and addiction called The Meadows in Wickenburg, Arizona. She provides some details on psychological issues in Chapter 6.

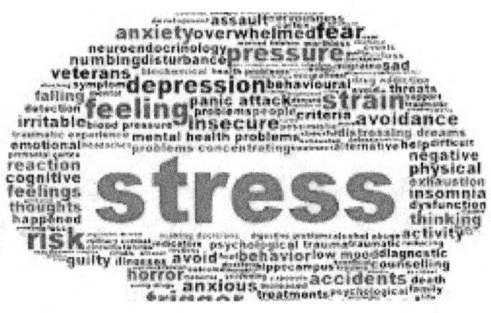

*Less Well-Known Risks*

The most obvious and well-known risk is aging. With the inevitability of your body getting older over time, you are nearly guaranteed to experience different types of pain. That doesn't mean that you have to resign yourself to it. The more you reduce risky behavior and actions, the healthier your back will be as you age. Is it easy - not until new behaviors become a habit. But it is definitely worth the time you put into changing your regular behaviors.

# Common Causes – Your Back's History

When you think of someone in their 40s rubbing a particular part of their back, that is the kind of pain that you can actually manage and heal. The pains of regular use are often from people *not* doing the things that they know they should be doing. Some pain is caused by an injury, like mine was when I was in high school. Sometimes that pain can be completely cured, although the areas around the injury will gristle and look a little rough in MRIs. Other pains are permanent and can always be a source of pain when triggered.

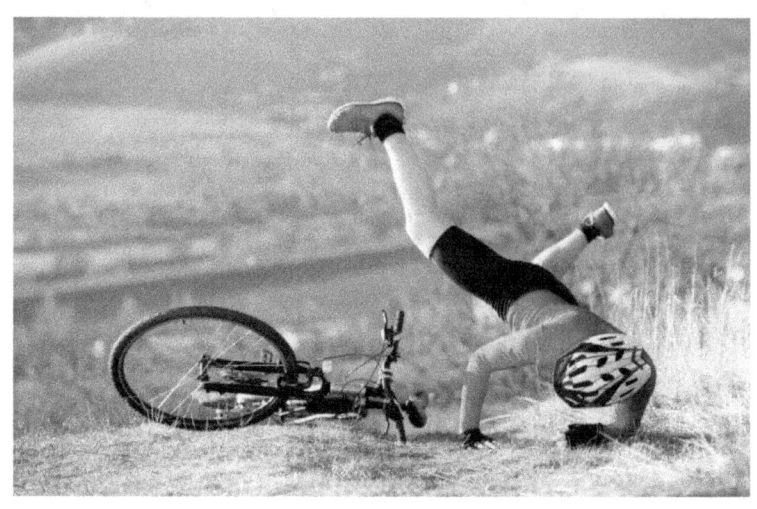

*Sport Injuries Are a Common Cause of Non-Genetic Back Pain*

This section delves into the kinds of things that are the most common contributors to back pain. Remember, these are different from risks because the pain is already there. The previous sections focused on things that you do that increase the likelihood that you will have back pain. This section focuses on reasons why you may be suffering now (not the reasons that you will suffer later).

## Genetics

Unfortunately, your genetics may make you predisposed to back problems. Taking care of yourself will significantly reduce a lot of the risks, but sometimes genetics make things a little more difficult for you. There are a whole host of genetic ailments that can cause back pain, and medical professionals are constantly researching new ailments and genetic connections to back problems.

According to one study conducted by King's College in London, researchers found a genetic connection to an increased likelihood of suffering from lower back pain. While everyone will suffer from the usual wear and tear, some people are actually more likely to have problems with their discs than others. By reviewing the MRI images from about 4,600 different individuals, researchers found that some people had a more rapid deterioration of their discs than others. They focused on lumbar disc degeneration, or LDD, and found that some of the participants had a faster rate of deterioration. We still have a long way to go to understand the problems, but there isn't much that can be done from a genetic perspective.

If you do have a genetic tendency to back problems, it is even more essential that you start to implement actions and activities that promote back health. By taking care of yourself when you are young, you can decrease the risk of some problems and slow down the rate of any problems that may present themselves later in life.

Other conditions, such as scoliosis, require intervention, depending on how severe they are. With many children going through regular checks at school to be examined for this condition, it is fairly well researched and understood. The actions that you can take are fairly well established to help you manage the problem. Skeletal irregularities are almost always genetic (although there are a few other things that can cause them).

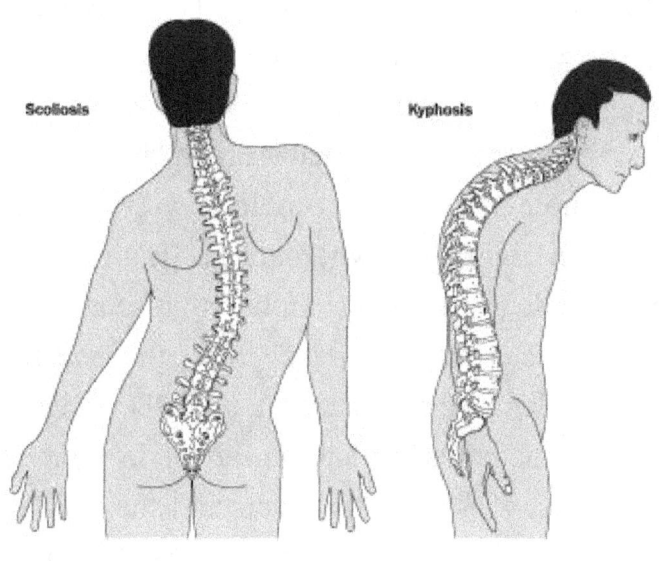

*Skeletal Irregularities and Anomalies Can Be the Main Problem Behind Your Back Pain*

As critical as it is, there is still so much that is unknown and debated about the back that it can be disheartening. Genetics is a particularly tricky area because so much is still up for debate. Some doctors do not believe in degenerative disorders, saying that problems always have a cause. However, there are degenerative disorders that are associated with other body parts, so it is very likely that problems are simply a lot harder to identify when they are in the back. It is certainly true that doctors tend to jump on the idea that a person is either imagining the pain or that they have a degenerative disorder without really taking the time to understand the source of the pain. Degenerative disorders tend to be genetic though, and there is very likely a small percentage of the population that is prone to more rapid spinal degeneration, just like with many other genetic ailments. It is certainly not something that should be a default diagnosis though. Even if you have a degenerative disorder, there are usually steps that you can take to slow the problem down.

It is possible that fibromyalgia and some of the only recently acknowledged ailments are genetic. There isn't nearly enough research or understanding of many disorders to know if they are genetic. Fibromyalgia does not just affect the back, nor does arthritis. The more research that is done on the old and new ailments, the more we will be able to do to treat the problems.

## Every Day Wear

Even if you have great genetics and don't suffer from an injury, you still have fairly good odds that you are going to have back pain as you age. A lot of your problems are going to stem directly from your choices and how you treat your back today. Here are some of the most common types of activities that you do that will almost certainly cause you pain down the road.

- Sitting for prolonged periods of time is always going to cause you pain later. It is almost safe to say that there are no exceptions to this. Even if you have phenomenal posture, sitting for hours is not good for your back. Sitting compresses the vertebrae, which is always bad. Most of us have stood up and felt stiff in all the wrong places. This is because of the way your brain communicates (or doesn't communicate) with your gluteus medius when you are sitting. Your gluteus medius works when you are walking; its primary purpose is to keep us balanced when we are walking as it provides support when we lift one foot from the ground. When you are sitting, you don't need any help with your balance. The gluteus medius is fully extended when you sit and affects all of the connecting muscles, and the longer you sit, the more all of these muscles are affected. After sitting for hours, the muscles will not work as effectively or efficiently. You will notice a strange sensation when you stand because you have been putting these muscles in an unhealthy position for far longer than they are meant to be in that position. Also the longer you sit, the worse your posture will get, which leads to the next point.

- Bad posture when sitting or reclining will do a lot of harm, particularly if you do it for hours at a time. You can also stand and walk with bad posture, which not only reinforces bad posture when you are sitting, but continues to hurt your spine and internal organs when you are supposed to be helping them.

- Lifting and reaching are activities that you do almost daily, and that can have its own negative effects. If you have to do these activities daily, you need to make sure that you are doing them in a way that is safe for your back and your legs. The tweaks and twinges of pain in those early days can quickly snowball into pains that get so much worse if you ignore them.

- Improper exercise, overdoing it, or doing exercises that intensify the pain are things that may seem more like isolated problems in the beginning. Maybe your lower back is a bit more sore after you start a new workout regimen, and it is hard to tell when it is a problem of overdoing it and when you are just pushing a little past your comfort zone. If the pain lasts for a few days, definitely consult your physician. Also, don't get complacent or sloppy in your routine. Ten years from now you should be focusing just as much on that yoga pose, set of repetitions, weightlifting, or whatever exercise it is that you are doing. Never get distracted or go into autopilot. That is exactly what can be among the worst kinds of wear and tear, as well as significantly increasing the odds that you will hurt yourself.

- Doing chores really is a collection of all of these, but it really needs to be specifically mentioned because it is while you are doing those chores that you are most likely to start noticing pain. It will probably start small, a small tweak in your back when you finish mowing. You rub it a little, and it feels alright after a few moments. Getting down on your knees to clean up spots, clean under furniture, or scrub the toilet will result in a lot of pain as you age, and you may not focus on your back because of the pain in your knees. When you are finishing your chores, take a moment to analyze your body, but particularly your back. If you find that it feels a bit sore, stretched, or has any kind of discomfort, you will need to be more aware of how you clean the next time. Find out what you did that could make your back feel that level of discomfort. It could be as easy as your posture, or it may be the way you stretched to reach into a corner. One of the most common problems is the way people stand. A proper hip hinge can signficiantly reduce stress on your back. When you stand, the hip hinge motion goes through your hip joints in an effort to keep your spine in a neutral position. All of the weight of your body is placed on your hips and legs instead of on your spine, which is exactly what you want to reduce the stress on your back, especially if you are suffereing from back pain. You should be keepng your back straight. An improper hip hinge will result in spine curvature, placing considerable stress almost exclusively on your back, and if you do this every time you stand, you are hurting your back several times a day, every day. I will go into how to do a proper hip hinge in a later chapter so that you can take better care of your back. If you would like, you can also watch videos on how to execute a proper hip hinge so that you can get started today. Simply being aware will help you to start changing bad habits and being more aware of what you are doing to cause yourself more stiffness or pain.

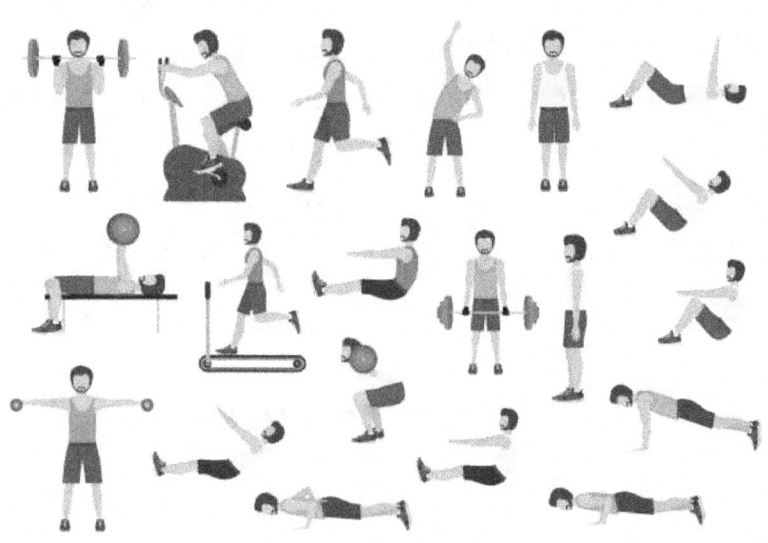

*Exercise Should Be Done Safely as Well as Regularly*

It is easy to go about your day, ignoring little pains and discomfort because we know that happens over time.

Don't.

As you continue to age, don't simply dismiss that pain. It probably won't become anything significant but, then again, it might. If you can save yourself even from mild pain later, it is always worth it.

## Injuries

Easily the most obvious type of back pain comes from an injury. These pains are impossible to miss and you know exactly what caused any problem you may have over the coming years. The more active you are, the more likely it is that you are going to do some kind of damage to your back.

The next chapter will go into the kinds of common injuries and the types of treatment that are likely to be required to help resolve or minimize the pain. If you have a specific injury that you know is causing your problems, or if you suspect it will cause problems down the road go ahead and read the next chapter to get started helping yourself today.

# CHAPTER 4

## Types of Injuries

Back pain is a kind of generic term that covers a whole host of possible injuries and problems. Your back is such a large part of your body and so integral in everything you do that pain seems like it is inevitable. As you will see in later chapters, back pain doesn't have to be a part of your fate. However, if you are already in your 30s or older, the damage up to this point is probably already starting to manifest itself in an occasional pain. Or maybe you have already begun calling in to work because the pain is a little too much to allow you to just push through the day.

Keep in mind that you should never be working through back pain unless you have no other choice, such as you are lost in the woods or are trapped on a desert island. Yes, these seem like extreme examples, but that is also the point.

Don't ignore the pain.

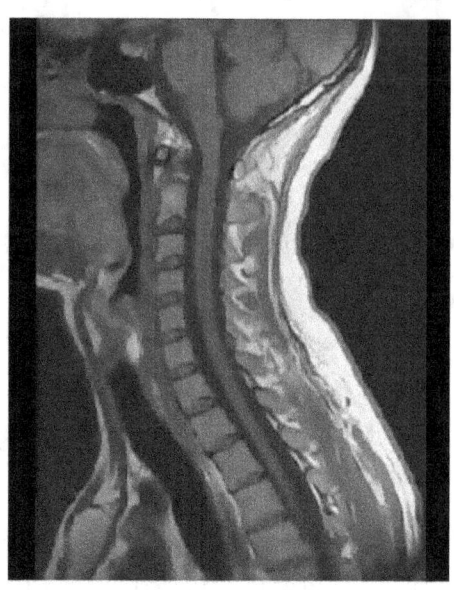

*Some Injuries Result in Obvious Issues*

Of course, if you are already experiencing pain, then you don't really care very much about what is causing your pain. You want to stop the pain, now. As difficult as it may be to focus on the solution, the best way to stop the pain is to treat the problem, and that means a lot more than just taking a couple of pills when your back really starts to hurt. With so many possible risks and ways to hurt your back, as easy as it may be to ignore the cause in favor of a quick fix, you really should understand the problem so that it doesn't happen again. There are three primary types of injuries that have very different types of pain:

- Injuries, such as a sports injury or from a car accident
- Post-surgical pain

- Chronic pain with no obvious source (you are unaware of any injury to the area, but it still hurts), is usually caused by the things you do every day

If you are reading this book and are worried that surgery is likely to be in your future, you should know that a lot of surgical procedures are not necessary. Because your back is so essential to every movement, if surgery is necessary you won't want to risk things getting worse. According to the UC Irvine Department of Orthopedic Surgery, only 5% of people who suffer from back pain require surgery. This is incredibly fortunate because most people who undergo surgery will suffer post-surgical pains, as well as being at an increased risk of becoming addicted to opioids. Surgery really is a last resort, so you may not need it.

What you will need to do is change how you treat your back. It is never too late to do that though. Even if you suffer from chronic pain, you can still help to alleviate the pain and learn how to adjust your habits to keep from constantly putting the same kind of strain on the areas that hurt.

There is always something you can do, and knowing the source of the pain will help you make the right decision about your care. That is what I hope to help you to do by the end of this book, as well as it being my goal for each patient who visits my clinic.

# Common Causes of Injury

Being an active person who participates in many outdoor activities, sports, and events is a great way to live. You are more likely to be healthy, but the additional wear and tear on your back from the activity can increase your likelihood of back issues. As I found out, you also do put yourself at risk of injuring your back or neck, and this can be extremely painful. The kinds of injuries that you are likely to sustain will depend on what your regular activities are. There are many more inherent risks to playing football than hiking. The kinds of pain you develop if you are a weekend warrior compared to a person who goes to the gym regularly is also going to vary significantly. A person who regularly stays active all week is going to experience fewer of the kinds of pains that result from being sedentary over the week and then cramming a lot of activity into the weekend. While the kinds of pain may vary, and the area of your back that is affected can be different based on your activity, there are only so many types of injuries that your back can sustain. It is when you actually damage your spine that you have a more intense and debilitating pain. These types of injuries can have more long-term effects.

Injuries typically result in the kind of back pain that will land you in a doctor's office. While it is possible that injuries to the spine can be alleviated and will largely heal without intervention, it is when you consider the long-term effects that you need to think about how to treat that part of your back.

Not all pain is intense the way mine was in high school or later in life. Sometimes it is just a tweak that causes discomfort.

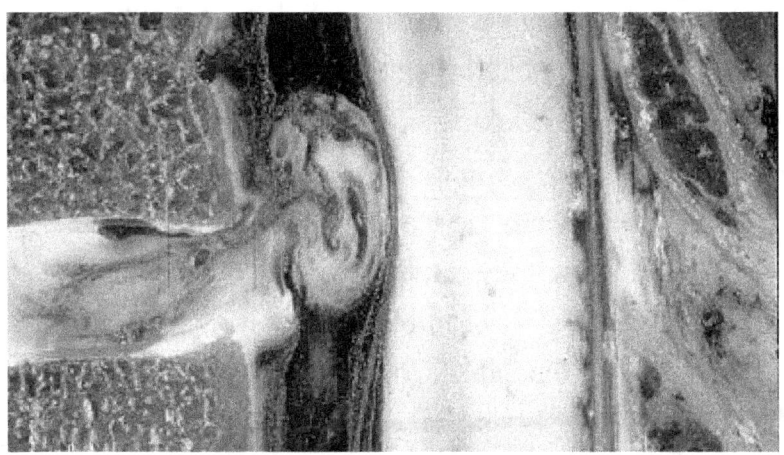

*Injuries Usually Include Your Discs and Surrounding Areas*

The following are the two most common types of back injury:

- Acute injuries – sudden movements or events that cause intense pain, and may include swelling and bruising around the area.

- Overuse or repetitive injuries – pain caused by overusing certain parts of your back or by repetitive motions that eventually cause pain.

If you are suffering from an injury, you know which one of the two ways you hurt your back, but that is also indicative of the kind of injury you sustained. The way to heal the injury is going to be different as well. What may not vary very much is how painful it can be. Acute injuries may cause immediate pain, but people call out of work far more often for injuries that are caused by overuse of the muscles in the back.

Acute Injuries

As I learned firsthand, acute injuries can be entirely disruptive, but all acute injuries are not like that. There was no bruising when I pinched a nerve, and the swelling was not obvious by simply looking at the site. With the back, most pains are not easily visible. The more serious problems are usually visible through the scans, which is probably why most people tend to think they can just wait to see if the injury heals. If you can't *see* that it is injured, it is easy to take a wait and see approach. Depending on the severity of the pain, sometimes it is obvious that you need to seek help sooner rather than later.

The kinds of injuries that often result from acute injuries include the following:

- Torn muscles or ligaments, usually classified as strains or sprains. They can be treated with home remedies, but will often require medical intervention to repair them.

- Injuries that compress the nerves of the lower back can be quite painful, although the pain may build to be more intense over time instead of all at once.

- Ruptured or torn discs are more common than most people realize. Larger tears can result in the soft tissue pushing out of the disc, and this is when you have a herniated disc. As the soft tissue pushes out of the disc, it can begin to build pressure on the nerve, which can lead to an incredible amount of pain. This is a problem that can become progressively worse, particularly if you have a small rupture that goes untreated. Typically, lower back pain is caused by ruptured or herniated discs.

- Pain cascading occurs when you sustain an injury and the injury begins to affect surrounding areas. Herniated discs will start to put pressure on other discs or the nerves in your spine. This pain can become quite intense. Torn discs also start to leak chemicals that can cause additional pain and discomfort. These chemicals affect the nerve fibers in the immediate area, and these fibers are very sensitive. When the chemicals start to affect the fibers, they can trigger swelling, which will further intensify the pain. The longer the discs leak, the more pain you will feel for a longer duration. Inflammation caused by the chemicals can last for weeks.

- Fractures or dislocation of the spine are the most serious types of injuries. If there is any question about whether a person's spine has been fractured or dislocated, you should never move that person. Any movements or changes in position can make the damage much more severe. Medical professionals should be the ones to stabilize the patient's body before it is moved. These are the kinds of injuries that can result in paralysis or death.

- There are many ways to sustain an acute injury, from skiing and playing rough sports to car accidents and daily exercise. You never know what will cause an acute injury because of how varied the reasons and injuries are. With just a simple motion, you may find yourself nearly incapacitated, and that can be very frightening.

## Overuse or Repetitive Injuries

The back isn't exactly known for these kinds of injuries. Typically, you would consider areas like the hand, wrist, or knee as locations that are more likely to sustain an injury through overuse or repetitive injuries. There are even a lot of different names for these kinds of injuries to other body parts, such as tennis elbow or carpel tunnel. Just because most people don't consider the back as a prime location for this type of problem though does not mean that it isn't. Given how much we use our back and how we move without even thinking about it, it really shouldn't come as a surprise. I think that it is likely that we just lump all of the problems with the back into a single category – back pain – instead of really figuring out what is wrong.

This will really work against you for injuries sustained through overuse and repetition though. Unlike acute injuries, overuse and repetition wear down a perfectly healthy back. The root cause is always you and your habits. There is no blaming other outside forces, which I've mentioned before and will go into in more depth later.

As if to make it seem less dangerous, there aren't any names for these kinds of injuries. To be fair, with causes as mundane as having bad posture when sitting or walking, sleeping on unsupportive furniture, or spending months or years weightlifting the wrong way, these kinds of injuries don't really require a name. That would really just call attention to the fact that it is something that you have been doing to yourself over time. I think this may actually be better in the long run. We overuse other body parts, and few body parts are nearly as crucial to us as our backs. By assigning names to the many different ways to injure yourself over time, I believe people would be more proactive in how they take care of their backs. This can only be better for the overall health of our backs.

The kinds of pains you get through overuse or repetition are typically less severe in the beginning. You will feel a spasm or a twitch in the muscles. You shake it off and keep going, only to feel it again a day or two later. Perhaps you wake up feeling stiffer than normal, and that keeps happening over time. There is a dull pain that you simply massage and then ignore, or you take a pain killer and don't change anything that you are doing.

And that is exactly what makes these kinds of injuries so risky. Never ignore pain. Your back is telling you that something needs to change – never ignore that. Perhaps it isn't as devastating in the early days as a herniated disc, but with time you are just scratching the scab and exacerbating the problem. In a year, five years, or a decade, you could find yourself in a much worse situation than many people with the acute injuries because you wanted to continue working through the pain instead of fixing the problem.

## When to See a Medical Professional

You definitely should not go a full three months dealing with the same pain. If your back does not start to feel better within a couple of weeks, you really need to make an appointment to start having the problem identified. The longer you go without getting proper treatment, the longer it is going to take to fix the problem. In many cases, reducing your activity, resting, and using normal home remedies will be adequate for duller pains and injuries that don't significantly interrupt your life.

Obviously, if you have suffered an acute injury you shouldn't wait too long, especially if the affected area is around the spine. These injuries seldom require surgery, but they may require you to change the way you do things to properly address the damage. You may need to have your spine realigned or take a couple of weeks when you are less active. Since many people won't do this without being told to, there is definitely a benefit from going to a medical professional. It is also good to make sure there isn't something more seriously wrong. Whiplash can take a while manifest itself, but when it does, the pain can be very intense. This is exactly why you should always see a physician after a car accident or an incident that jolted your body.

If you suspect that there might be damage to the spine, always seek medical assistance. Some of the problems may be small but will become progressively more painful and damaging as time goes by.

# Post-Surgery

Surgery is almost always a last resort because of the associated risks. Your back can take a lot of stress and tension and end up being perfectly alright if you give it the proper care. The biggest problem is often that people simply don't give their back the amount of rest that is required for it to heal. Medication has its place, but it is not a cure all – most of the time medicine is just a way to temporarily relieve pain. You should not be using medication to mask pain or to make it easier to keep doing whatever you have been doing that caused the problem. If your pain persists or if the damage is extensive, then surgery could be required. Your doctor will take many factors into consideration before making a recommendation to go through with surgery.

### Surgery Considerations

I just said that medicine is not a cure all – the truth is that medicine isn't any kind of healer. When a doctor changes your medication, what you should know is that it is never meant to help heal your back. Back pain medication is pretty much just a way to minimize pain so that you can continue to function. Most types of back pain are not caused by anything that can be cured with medication. It is estimated that

Americans spend more than $86 billion a year because of back pain – that is a lot of money for something that is not meant to cure the problem. There are a few conditions that medication will help, but the vast majority of back pain is related to way that you use your back, which is why you ultimately have to start learning how to do things differently after giving your back some time to rest.

If your back is seriously injured, whether through an accident or through sustained over use, here are the things that doctors will take into account before recommending surgery.

- The root cause of the pain is the most significant consideration. Most injuries can be treated through less drastic means, so the doctor needs to spend time determining exactly what is wrong. Only severe injuries will require surgery, conditions that cannot be healed in any other way.

- Determining the risks is the next major consideration. With more severe injuries that have an associated risk of paralysis, back surgery is almost certainly going to be required. But most other problems, even herniated discs, usually won't require surgery. Surgery should never be used like medicine – there are better ways to manage pain that are far less risky. With the potential for the surgery to cause worse pain or injury, you only want to select it as a final solution, never jump into it instead of taking other less invasive methods to fix the problem for less critical injuries.

Once you have had back surgery, you will need to go through physical therapy. Back surgery is incredibly invasive and you will require weeks to months to get back to where you were before you underwent the surgery. Your back is critical to everything you do, so you will be out of commission for a while after the surgery.

Some back surgeries fail. It is nearly as difficult to research as back pain, failed back surgery syndrome (FBSS) can be the end result of surgery. FBSS occurs when the performed surgery does not eliminate or minimize the pain a patient experiences in the lumbar portion of their back. According to data compiled by Baber and Erdek (2016), nearly a third of patients who had surgery on their lumbar stenosis suffered from more pain a year after the surgery. Based on a study by Parker, et. al. (2015), researchers found that between 5 and 36% of patients experience pain within two years of the surgery. According to P. F. Ullrich Jr. (2004), the amount of time required to recover from spine fusion surgery is between 3 months and a year. There are many variables, and with how invasive surgery can be, most physicians will recommend other methods of relief and will give patients between 6 to 12 months to see if they can get relief through these other methods before resorting to surgery.

Given how costly they can be and how painful the recovery process is, there are many good reasons that surgery is often a last resort. Back pain can be distracting, but it is rarely a reason to undergo surgery without trying virtually everything else first. The next couple of chapters will go into this in more depth, looking at your options, from medications to alternative treatments, such as physical therapy, acupuncture, chiropractic, and regenerative medicine. You also need to understand the root cause of the pain before undergoing surgery. If the root cause is not properly identified, then surgery will do far more harm than good.

## Quick Test

If your doctor is considering surgery, always get a second opinion (unless you are at risk of paralysis or after a critical, acute injury).

There is also something you can try yourself. It could be best to consult with a specialist, like a regenerative medicine specialist or a functional rehab therapist. Most people fail to take the most critical step of letting their back rest when they start to feel minor pain, and that is what ultimately makes things worse or fail to improve. Yes, you may love jogging, but if it is hurting you, then you need to take a couple of weeks off. Don't entirely stop exercising, you can still walk, but don't over work your back. Spend more time being less aggressively active. The time that you used to spend jogging or going to the gym can be used to take nice walks instead. Don't sit or lie down for hours at a time – this is also detrimental to your back. You don't need to become sedentary; you just need to put less strain on your back. It is a delicate balance between reducing your activity and ensuring that you are active enough not to place more pressure on your back. Remember, being too inactive puts just as much stress on your back as trying to maintain all of your usual activities.

Keep in mind that your response to an acute injury should not be treated like this. You need to see a physician to start analyzing the problem. There are too many potentially damaging injuries that will be exacerbated by being too sedentary. Resting can sometimes do more harm than good. A physician can determine what the problem is and what the best path forward is.

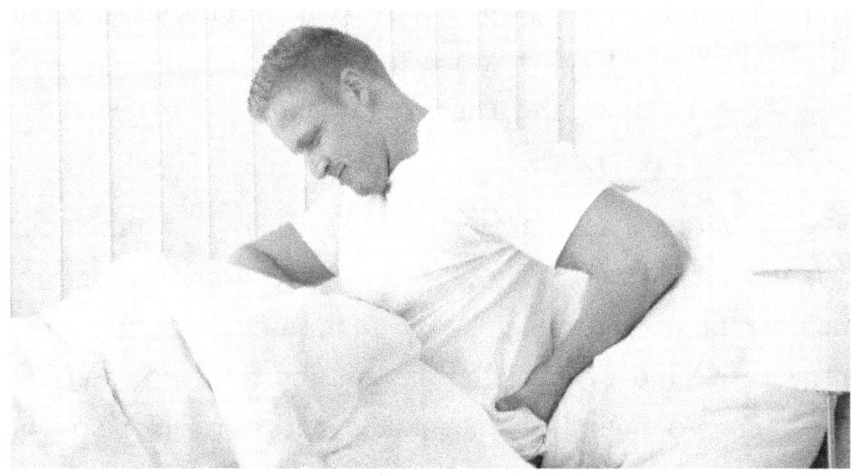

*Rest Your Back*

In most cases, you already know what measures will help, and surgery is almost certainly not one of those ways to help your back. Remember, only about 5% of people who report back pain resort to surgery. Do the things that you think are inconvenient but that will help your back because those changes are something you will have to do after back surgery, and you will be far more limited in what you can do immediately after surgery. It's a matter of relenting and realizing that you have more time in your schedule to do the right thing than being bed ridden and suffering as you try to recover.

## Chronic Pain

Chronic back pain is a recurring pain that is still present three months after your back first begins to hurt. This can be caused by an injury, but it can also be caused by regular wear and tear on your back. Nor do you have to feel it all of the time, but if the same part of your back continues to hurt at least intermittently for more than three months, that is considered chronic pain. The pain does not have to be intense either.

Chronic back pain can be caused by disc problems, overuse, repetition, lack of rest, strains, sprains, or any number of other problems. By continuing to execute the provocative movements that are causing the pain, you are definitely prolonging it. It is possible that your back pain will continue after treatments because you aren't giving your back the proper considerations and alternative movements to keep from triggering the pain. Since we use our backs for nearly every movement, it can be very difficult to rest as much as we need to. Unfortunately, there could be other reasons why the pain does not disappear. An estimated 20% of people who report having acute back pain develop chronic back pain following the initial event. Their pain is still present a year later, making it very difficult to resume their normal lives. I've seen this many times, and know that it can become very frustrating, as well as painful.

One of the greatest risks of chronic back pain is the risk of becoming addicted to the pain medication. People can begin to believe that they simply cannot eliminate the pain, and think that they will need to continue to take medication to manage it. This is a large contributor to the current Opioid Crisis in the US, and it is something that is absolutely not as essential as people may think. There are many other options that can help you manage, reduce, or eliminate chronic pain that have none of the risks of pain killers. The next couple of chapters will go into this in more detail. For now, just know that chronic pain has a much higher risk of drug addiction because people accept that medicine is a part of their life – something that no one should ever accept. Chronic back pain isn't like a disease that requires medication; it is pain that is letting you know that you need to do something differently. Back pain medicine is largely pain relief medicine, and that is making it possible for you to do the exact opposite of what you should be doing. Instead of minimizing or stopping the provocative motions that are causing the pain, you are masking the pain so that you can continue with those movements. This not only exacerbates the pain and problem, it means that you will suffer more pain once the medication wears off since you have been using your back instead of resting it.

Medical and surgical treatments may also result in chronic back pain, particularly if your back does not heal properly. There are risks associated with surgery, but as I can attest, not all treatments work either. What I had was not chronic back pain since I was mostly healed within a few weeks of starting treatment with my father's chiropractor friend. However, had I not found the solution, I could easily have become someone who suffered from chronic back pain. Since 1990, the number of people who have reported chronic back pain has gone from being the sixth to the third most burdensome health condition in the US. The only two conditions that cause greater concern are ischemic heart disease and chronic obstructive pulmonary disease. Note, this is for diseases that either contribute to higher mortality rates or poor health.

Chronic back pain is less common than most kinds of pain and it can indicate that there is something more seriously wrong with your back. This is particularly difficult to treat because the reasons for chronic back pain go well beyond what most people associate with back pain. Treatment isn't as easy as being more aware of your posture or making sure you don't sit for too long (though these measures can help some) and surgery may not even be an option for these possible causes.

While injuries are a large contributor to chronic back pain, they are not the only causes. Ailments like fibromyalgia are not back specific, but they can cause you significant and constant pain in your back. Arthritis can also contribute to back pain, and while it is typically specific to a particular area, it is not easy to treat. These kinds of problems are the most difficult to treat because there really isn't a solution beyond simply managing the pain.

It can be very difficult to diagnose the root cause because of all the potential contributors to chronic back pain. If you experience an acute injury, it will be easier to start to understand the problem, but for most other types of chronic back pain, the cause will be less easy to identify. Keeping a journal of the kinds of activities that trigger the pain, the times of day or year, the intensity of the pain, the things that alleviated the pain, or anything else that you can record can be helpful in better understanding the pain so that you and your physician can find the best way to start to treat it. Images of your back may help, particularly if the pain is caused by a tumor or other problem that you may not anticipate, but often images are only marginally helpful. We all do things that affect our backs, so anomalies and gristle are going to be visible, and those are not necessarily a sign of the problem. Often these anomalies and gristle are actually fine, and the problem is something that you cannot see in an image or scan. By keeping records of the events around the pain, you can start to help identify the problem.

# CHAPTER 5

# What Medicine Has to Offer

With an estimated 80% of adults stopping by the doctor's office to get advice about their back pain at least once in their lives, there is an enormous market for dealing with this particular malady. Considering that there are a plethora of over the counter pain killers, it is easy to see why these adults are looking for something a little stronger. Even for people who don't want a stronger pain killer, taking pills every day or every time they experience back pain is not a way to resolve the issue. No matter what part of you hurts, pain killers are always supposed to bring a temporary relief – you aren't supposed to make them a part of the daily routine to manage pain.

There are some ailments that make it necessary to use pain killers daily, such as arthritis. However, these are the exceptions, and not the rule. You want to manage pain with pain killers temporarily, not rely on pain killers to help you get through your day, every day. Ultimately, the goal is to get rid of the problem, and not to just treat the pain. It is why you need to find the source instead of working through the pain.

Back pain isn't like a cold, a virus, asthma, or allergies. The problem is almost certainly caused by damage to the back (with the genetic problems being an exception), and that means that the way to heal the injury is going to be through your actions; not constant medication. You simply need medication to help you alleviate the pain so that you can focus on other things until the root problem is addressed.

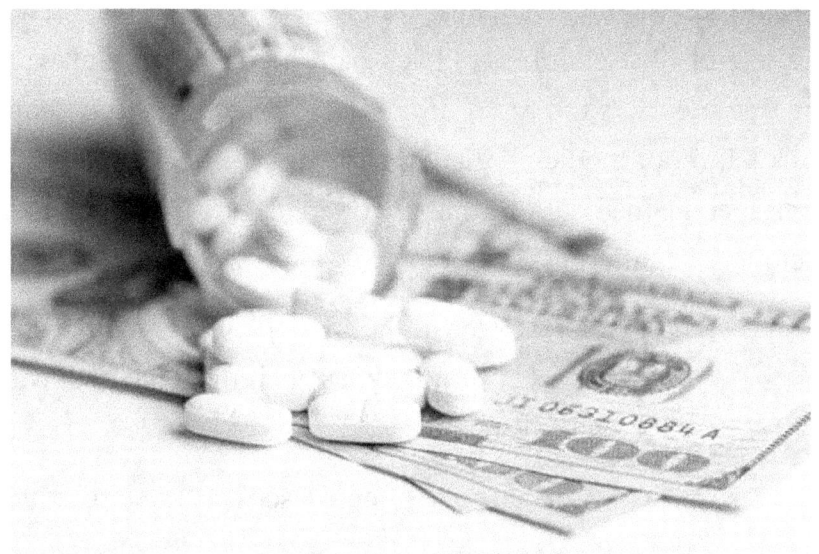

Medications definitely have a place for short term tweaks and strains that just require you to be a little less active for a few days. For pain that is a little more intense, stronger types of medicine can be very helpful in getting through the problem until you've learned how to bend differently, keep a good posture, and whatever other corrections you need to make until they become a habit. However, you never want to become dependent on drugs because of the negative problems that come with back pain medications.

# The Different Kinds of Back Pain Medications

The thing to keep in mind about back pain medications is that these medicines really aren't specific to the back. Yes, the title of this section says back pain medications, but what the title means is the types of medicine prescribed to manage back pain, not medicine that is made just for backs. The non-back specific medications that are often used to treat back pain include four different types.

- Nonsteroidal anti-inflammatory drugs (NSAIDs) are the most common types of medicine to deal with back pain.

- Muscle relaxers are often prescribed to help reduce back tension.

- Opioids are prescribed to help manage more intense back pain and they target the nerve receptors to alleviate that pain.

- Antidepressants are not commonly associated with back pain, but they are prescribed in some cases to help manage the pain, even if a patient is not exhibiting any symptoms of depression.

These medications can be quite effective when it comes to helping you continue your regular routine, but they are never meant to be the cure for the problem. If you continue to suffer from pain in the same location in your back, you need to visit a doctor instead of thinking that the problem will eventually disappear. Dulling or reducing the pain you feel means that you are more likely to continue with the provocative motions that are causing the pain, which is exactly what you shouldn't be doing. Consider these kinds of medications as the short-term solution you use to keep you going while taking the necessary steps to determine the cause of the pain. You will need to treat the problem, and it is not done through medication.

## NSAIDs

Essentially, these are the over-the-counter medicines that may be recommended to you, but you probably already have some of these in your home . Their primary purpose is right there in the name – they reduce swelling and inflammation. They also reduce how much pain you feel around the affected area. You can take as much of the medication as you feel you need within the recommended dose over the course of the day. Typically, you shouldn't take more than 2 pills or capsules every four hours. If you want to take less than that, you can without worrying about adverse effects.

Since they are easy to access, people often become dependent on NSAIDs, and that can cause a myriad of other health issues. The following are some of the most common problems associated with reliance on NSAIDs:

- Cramps and stomach pain
- Bleeding

- Ulcers
- Kidey damage

This is why you have to be particularly careful when you start to use any medication. Don't let the relief that you get allow you to postpone resolving the real problem. Becoming reliant on the drug is a problem on its own, which means you will be dealing with your current problem and another one later on because you never addressed the root cause of your pain.

## Muscle Relaxers

The name of the medication says exactly what this medication does. By targeting the central nervous system, these medications can help relieve the pain that is affecting the muscles. If you experience muscle spasms, then your doctor may recommend muscle relaxers to help you relax. They tend to be very effective, and often you only need a half or a quarter of a pill at a time. It can reduce pain by making the muscles relax, which can be required since tense muscles can intensify the pain. This type of medication is often used in conjunction with other treatments as it can help you to move your back and legs with greater ease.

If you are prescribed muscle relaxers, you should plan to stay at home since they are known for making people drowsy. You should not use them when you are at work, before driving, or when you need to be alert. Once you take them, you are likely to just sit around and rest or fall asleep. Muscle relaxers do not just relax the back, but they relax all of the muscles in your body. This can be great when you are in intense pain or if you have been too tense for extended periods of time because of pain, just be aware that a small amount is all it takes for most people to feel out of it.

## Opioids

I will go into this class of medications in more detail in the next chapter because there are many ramifications to using opioids. There is no doubt that in terms of doing what they should, opioids are extraordinarily effective. Medications like oxycodone and hydrocodone can keep your receptors from registering the pain, but that isn't always a good thing. Instead of developing a reliance on medication (as can happen with NSAIDs), opioids can lead to addiction.

Using opioids is not a problem as long as they are used while addressing the real problem and are used only for a short period of time. They should never be a first resort, but a last resort. If your physician jumps to this as a solution, find someone else because the risks for using opioids are very high. Opioids aren't as risky as surgery, and you will likely use opioids before surgery will be considered, but it is one of the last things to try before surgery. And you should always start using them while you are being treated for the real problem, not as a way of managing pain on its own.

## Antidepressants

Doctors may decide to prescribe antidepressants for some lower back pain, regardless of a person's mental state.

One of the most common antidepressants used for back pain is duloxetine. The reason why some physicians opt to prescribe an antidepressant is because they are not addictive. This kind of medication works directly on the brain to suppress the way it senses pain. Research is still being conducted to understand how the medication helps, but antidepressants work with fewer long-term risks compared to opioids. However, they do not have an immediate effect on the pain, so you will need to give the drug some time to take effect before you will start to feel the pain less intensely.

While they are not addicting, there are other side effects associated with antidepressants, including the following:

- Constipation or nausea
- Sleepiness
- Shifting weight
- Sweating and shaking
- Dry mouth
- Blurred vision

The side effects will vary based on which antidepressant you are taking, so you will need to find out exactly what to watch for before starting to use any antidepressant. Your doctor can also change the prescription if one isn't working.

# The Good

Trying to get anything done when your back hurts is only slightly easier to do than if you have a headache. When your back hurts, nearly everything you do can be uncomfortable at the best and downright painful at the worst. You may end up sitting in a position that is really bad for your body to try to minimize the pain, or change the way you walk, causing different problems, all to compensate for the pain in your back. Taking NSAIDs to reduce that pain is completely understandable in the early days.

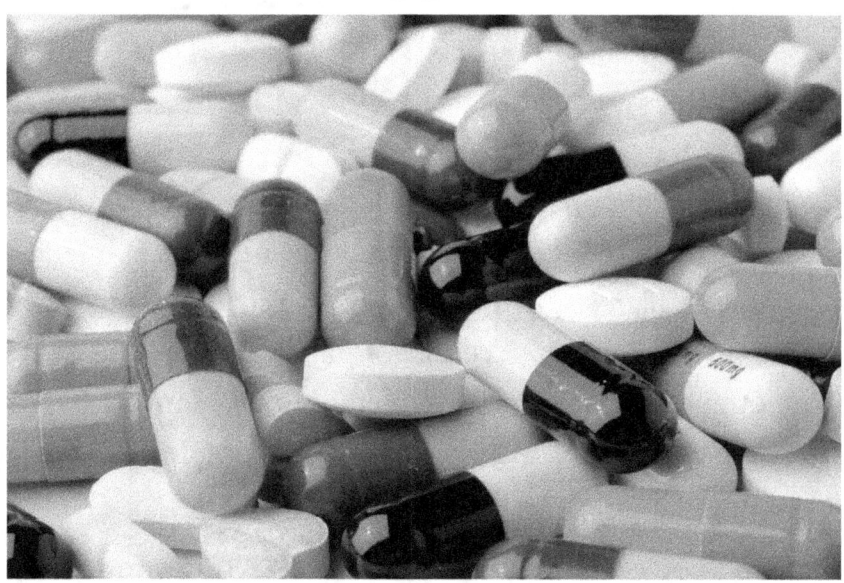

For injuries, medication can help you to adjust while you are undergoing treatment or rehab to fix the problem. Being able to continue to function or to have something that allows you to go through rehab is essential to the recovery. Bed rest can be detrimental because most of the time it will do more damage than good. With so many people reporting back pain as we become more sedentary, too much inaction is probably one of the initial contributing factors. You should be more active if this is part of the reason for your pain, not less. You just need to be more careful not to do anything that puts additional strain or stress on the affected area.

Medication allows you to continue or resume activities with more focus than if the pain is not reduced. Being able to function is an essential part of the recovery, and medication makes that possible. Just as you would take medication for a headache or serious injury, back pain medication is incredibly effective when used responsibly.

## The Bad

There are many potential downsides to back pain medications, with a reliance on them being one of the most common problems. It is far too common for people to reach for a bottle and to pop a couple of pills and then keep going like nothing is wrong – it is something that many of us are guilty of doing. And that on its own is problematic for a number of reasons.

As you get accustomed to taking NSAIDs, you develop a tolerance to them, which means you need to take more pills for them to be effective. Your body is not meant to be constantly processing pain killers. It is trying to tell you that there is something wrong, and you are responding by silencing your body instead of addressing the problem. Remember, none of these medications are a cure for the problem. They are simply a way of addressing the pain so that you can keep going – you need to find out what the actual problem is though. With such an easy solution available that will probably work for a while, it is easy to think that the problem isn't that severe. The longer you put off finding out the cause and continue to function without trying to remediate the behaviors that are causing or exacerbating the issue, the more harm you are doing to your back.

If your back is hurting and there hasn't been a single event that could have caused the injury, it means that your regular activities are the problem, whether it is your posture, sedentary days, over active weekends, or improper lifting. If you are dulling the pain, you are making it easier to continue to execute the movements that are detrimental, the kinds of movements that your back is trying to warn you about. The longer you take NSAIDs instead of seeking help, the more damage you could be doing to your back. This means that more serious treatments may be the required by the time you get around to finally seeking treatment. You have to address the problem, not use medication to help yourself ignore it. Pain is there for a reason, and should be taken seriously.

There are side effects that are associated with all of the different medications. Also, everyone is different, and how your body will react to a prescription medication is not entirely predictable. Muscle relaxers pretty much make it difficult to do anything. From personal experience, I can say that taking muscle relaxers can make it difficult to do anything for 24 to 48 hours. It felt like my head was stuffed with cotton and my ability to rationalize was negatively affected for a couple of days. This is not a great state to be in on a regular basis. Depending on the severity of the pain, you probably won't need to take them daily. For me, they were a way of relaxing the muscles in my back when I had built up too much stress and made the muscles too tense and could not relax the muscles myself, which triggered another pain in my back. I didn't need the medication every day, and rarely took two doses within a week. Still, I really did not like what the medicine did to my cognitive abilities. The best recommendation is to take them at night when you won't be going out or need to be alert.

Both opioids and antidepressants have a long list of possible side effects, with opioids having the additional risk of addiction. These possible side effects do make them much more dangerous, and are something that you need to take into account and discuss with your physician before you take them. Both of these medications can also affect cognitive abilities, which means you need to learn how you are affected after taking them before you plan to drive or do anything that requires you to be alert (such as driving). Some antidepressants can also cause depression in the beginning, which is why you have to be very careful about taking them. With either of these drugs, you will need to stay in touch with your doctors about any problems or side effects that you experience after taking the medication. People are also closely monitored after taking opioids and antidepressants because of the side effects. Neither drug is meant to be a long-term solution either, just a way to help you resume doing normal tasks as much as possible. It is also possible that you will suffer from itching or hives if you take opioids, which means that you are trading pain for a different kind of discomfort.

Opioids are often recommended for acute pain from an injury and after surgery. It is estimated that up to 70% of people who report back pain are prescribed opioids, and that is without a doubt far too many people taking something that they probably don't need. If your pain is so intense that you need something that strong, you have put off going to the doctor for far too long. If your physician does not try other medications and treatments first, you need to change your physician because opioids are far too potent to be an early option. If you suffer from a serious injury and are hospitalized, that is about the only reason I can think of when opioids would need to be given – and even then, it really depends on what is wrong. As intense as my pain was in high school, opioids were never something that should have been considered. The treatment I received from our family friend was the real solution, and then other less addictive pain killers were more than enough medication to help manage the pain while my back was convalescing.

# Medication Addiction and Reliance

Easily one of the worst side effects of any back-pain medication, addiction is on a different level than the other potential problems. Antidepressants won't lead to addiction, but the other three types of medications could become something you rely on or are addicted to, which is counter to what the drugs should do. Medication is meant to help you return to normal, not require you to keep taking it. The next chapter addresses this problem in more detail, but opioid addiction has ballooned into a national crisis as it damages communities across the US. The repercussions from addiction are far worse than most types of back pain. It is a risk that is a potential problem with most types of prescription medications, and the risk of addiction is something that needs to be taken into consideration before you start taking any potentially addictive prescriptions.

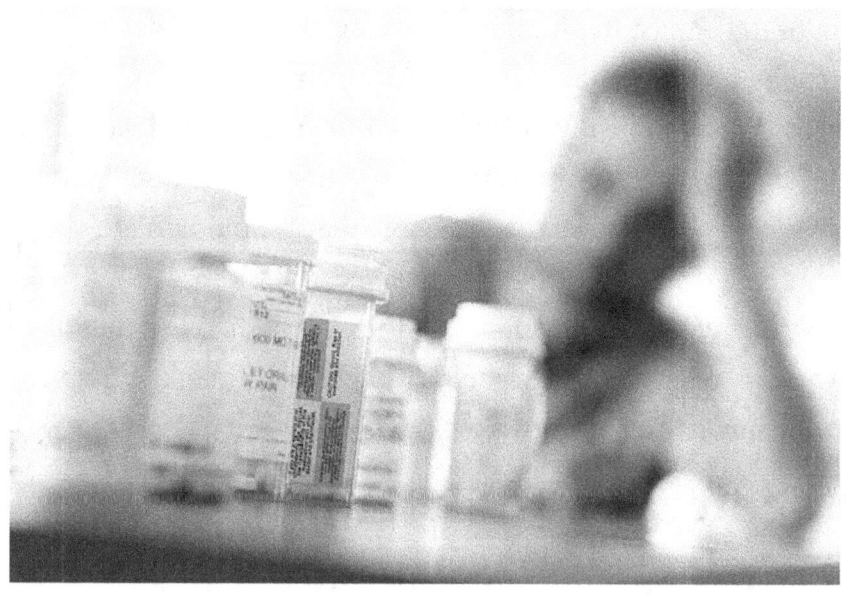

*Addiction Is a Serious Problem That Can Be More Detrimental than the Initial Problem*

You aren't likely to get addicted to most types of NSAIDs, but you may become reliant on them, which is also very unhealthy. Taking any medication for long periods of time can have some severe health effects.

There are only a few instances when the patient will need to continue to take medication for long periods of time. With a vast majority of people reporting back pain at least once in their life, you don't want to be someone who relies on any medication (and certainly don't want to risk addiction) for the rest of your life. You need to fix the problem and stop using drugs as soon as possible.

# How I Help Wean Patients away from a Reliance on Medicine

Since medication is not the solution to the problem (it is just a band aid), my clinic focuses on the problem and helping patients to fix it. Of course, there will be times when medicine is necessary, but those days are few and far between. Over time, change of diet, exercise, and a healthier lifestyle will make it clear that medicine was never a part of the solution. In the short term though, what you need is a peek into what life could be like if the root cause is treated. My education has been dedicated to the many new ways of looking at the most common back problems and providing an actual solution. Whether that means injections, acupuncture, or something else, we can determine what approach is right for your specific problem. We also take the time to assess the pain so that we have an idea of what the pain triggers are. That way we can make recommendations on things you can do differently without exacerbating the problem.

I know that seeing results is what ultimately leads to people taking a different approach and being more optimistic about the chance that they can actually remove or significantly reduce the pain. Making sure that my patients start to experience what life could be like is what really makes it worthwhile, and why I am more than happy to continue my education. There are always new methods that might offer a better way to treat a problem.

# CHAPTER 6

# Trauma, Mental Health, and the Opioid Crisis

One of the few perceived problems in the US today that people do not dispute is the Opioid Crisis. According to the US Health Resources and Services Administration, more than 130 people die every day because of an opioid or opioid-related overdose. This is a staggering number that is gaining the attention of politicians today as the demand for change becomes increasingly louder. A large part of the problem is the large number of people dealing with chronic pain, and pain in the lower back is one of the most common reasons people seek pain medication. The other major part of the problem is the willingness of doctors to prescribe opioids to help manage pain. Often the medication is prescribed with little or no attempt to resolve the problem that is causing the pain.

Opioids and prescription medications that contain opioids are incredibly addictive, which makes them a dangerous medication to prescribe without first exploring the use of other, less dangerous drugs. Doctors really should not be jumping to strong pain killers so quickly. There has been a lot of speculation and accusations of doctors getting benefits for prescribing these drugs, which has contributed to the overuse of opioids and the resulting increase in the numbers of the addicted.

I'm not going to speculate or go into the details of the practices of pharmaceutical companies and doctors because, ultimately, I want to help people learn to fix the problems. All opioids do is mask the pain. They aren't a long-term solution and they are not something I am going to recommend to my patients. My interest in discussing the opioid crisis is to highlight that the focus for back pain (and pain in general) has really gone awry, contributing to a serious health crisis in the US. Understanding the problems with the current general methods of dealing with back pain can help you make better decisions in how to manage your own back pain. The main go-to option is currently a dangerous medicine that is not necessary for most people. I want to help you understand why I make my recommendations and how they differ from the current norms. If you understand the risks and current state of the most common treatment, I hope to persuade you that other methods are much better suited to helping you to not only manage the pain, but to eliminate the root cause of the pain.

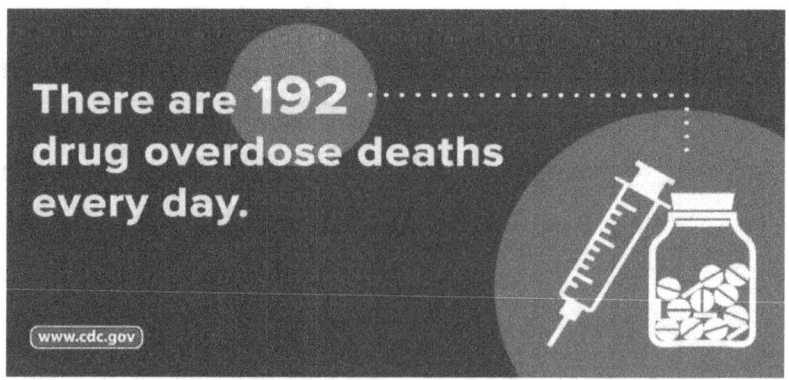

# A Brief History – How We Got Here

The Opioid Crisis has actually been going on for a lot longer than most people realize. Toward the end of the 1990s, pharmaceutical companies were trying to get more medications on the market, specifically medicines that included opiates. The effects of this ingredient were not unknown in the medical community as places like opium dens had been popular for several centuries. There were certain risks that were well known regarding opiates and the medical community was initially hesitant to prescribe any medication that included such a potentially addictive ingredient. Upon the assurance from many of the pharmaceutical companies that their medications were not as potentially dangerous or as addictive as the ingredient in its raw form was, the medical community began to prescribe the new medications.

Initially, the prescriptions were written for more serious pains. However, this quickly changed and physicians began to prescribe these strong pain killers for less critical pain, such as lower back pain and chronic pain. Over the next decade, these highly addictive drugs were prescribed for a host of pains, even minor ones, and little monitoring was done by physicians or pharmaceutical companies to ensure that patients were not becoming addicted. Within a decade, drugs that included opiates were being misused and over prescribed, leading to patients becoming reliant on the medication to just get through the day. Since physicians and doctors had become accustomed to prescribing opioid pain relievers, they would provide prescriptions for refills long after the patient should have stopped using the drug. Patients who had become addicted were able to seek out a new doctor to continue the prescription. Some patients even resorted to stealing the medication from family and friends because of how often opioids were prescribed for even minor pains.

Between 1999 when opiates were being prescribed as pain killers and 2017 when the epidemic could no longer be ignored, over 700,000 people in the US died from overdoses. In 2017 alone, 70, 200 people died from drug overdoses; of that estimate, more than 65% died from overdosing on opioids (47,600). This does include illegal drugs, such as heroin, but because of the fact that prescriptions include the same ingredients as the illegal drug, they are categorized together. Some people who become addicted to pain killers begin taking heroin because of the similarity in the effects. In 1999, opioid related overdoses were not nearly as common; by 2017, the increased number of people who died by overdosing on this particular drug was 6 times higher than when opioids first became a common prescription.

According to the US Centers for Disease Control and Prevention, there were three waves of increased opioid related deaths between 1999 and 2017.

- As the prescriptions became more common at the end of the 1990s, there was a significant increase in the number of deaths related to the increased use. Prior to this, the number of opioid related deaths had been on the decline as heroin had seen a decrease in its use.

- The next wave of increased opioid related deaths started during 2010. During this time, the rise of overdoses was related to the over-prescription of heroin-based drugs. Considering the fact that the use of the illegal drug had been in the decline, this was an unpleasant surprise that caused the medical profession and lawmakers to begin to take notice of how prevalent opioids had become in the lives of average Americans. They were being forced to acknowledge the potential dangers of the legal prescriptions which were clearly being prescribed at rates that far outweighed their need or recommendations.

- The third wave began just three years later in 2013 when there was a substantial rise in overdoses from illicitly-manufactured fentanyl. These drugs had seen a rise in use as an alternative to heroin and prescription drugs. This remains a problem today as the people who make these illegal drugs are still changing their production methods and products. Perhaps the greatest concern is that these drugs are being combined with the other types of illegal opioids and other drugs, such as cocaine. This makes them a particularly potent drug. With a large number of people dependent on opioid prescriptions now being cut off, there is real concern about how many people will turn to these newer, more powerful, and more dangerous opioids.

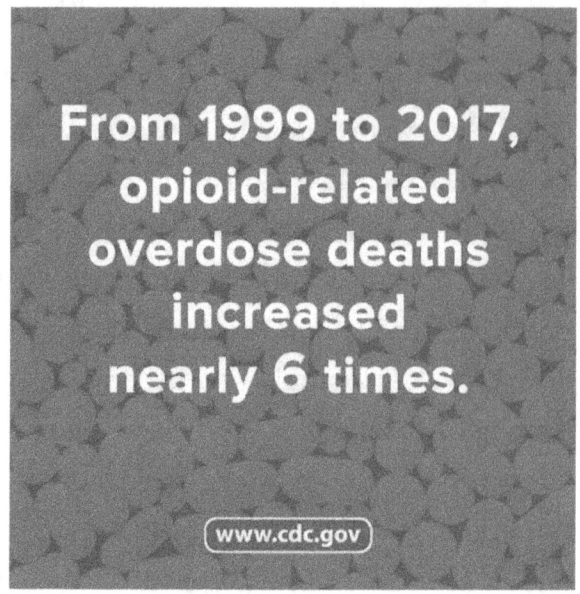

Not all of the problems are related to overdoses though. Simply being addicted has taken a significant toll on those who have been prescribed opioid medications. During 2017, an estimated 1.7 million Americans reportedly suffered from disorders from prescription opioids alone, including problems stemming from authorized use.

# Managing Chronic Pain

There are many problems with the use of opioids and opioid-related drugs to try to manage pain. However, the risks are particularly high for people who suffer from chronic pain as they will likely require more time to address the problem that is causing the pain. Some of the people who suffer from chronic pain will continue to suffer for the rest of their lives, which makes them at higher risk of addiction to the prescription drugs.

People who suffer from chronic pain should be offered other, less potentially dangerous means of managing their pain. Depending on the intensity and duration of the pain, the mild over-the-counter pain relievers could be adequate to help them through the worst of the pain. People who suffer from arthritis or fibromyalgia can turn to these kinds of pain medications without the risk of addiction. It is important to be careful not to become reliant on over-the-counter pain relievers though as the body cannot process the drugs every day for years without the serious risk of causing other problems.

Those who are suffering chronic pain from an injury or other problem often do not need opioid medications either as opioids never address the real problem.

The only time I feel it is a good idea to recommend these drugs is during hospital visits or for patients who will be under the watchful eye of a nurse or doctor for the duration of the prescription. It should *only* be used in conjunction with actual treatment methods that address the root cause, and never as a way of avoiding pain. You will use your back for everything you do, so to help you rehabilitate or overcome severe pain while trying to return to your more normal routines, you have to learn how to treat your back better. Hiding the pain just leads to worse pain and more serious issues over time. Whether or not the pain in your back is the result of an injury or normal wear-and-tear, you have to change your behavior to really recover. We all do things that we know are a bad idea, and even something as apparently innocuous as slouching can cause long-term detrimental effects on your back.

And to me, this is the hidden danger behind using many different kinds of medications to mask the pain, particularly something as potent as an opioid. Most of us have the problems we have *because* we keep working through the pain. It's not only foolish, but self-destructive. My problems with NSAIDs is only when people begin to rely on them. If you take them often, you will develop a tolerance to NSAIDS, making them ineffective when you actually need them. Once you develop this tolerance, your physician is going to prescribe something a bit stronger to help you. Obviously this is not how you want to spend the rest of your life, taking increasingly stronger and stronger medicines to manage the pain.

Remember that the goal is to eliminate the problem, not to push through the resulting pain and make the situation worse.

# Treating a Symptom – Not the Problem

This is something that I have frequently mentioned because it is critical to understand that back pain medication is not a cure – it does not treat the problem. The point of back pain medication is not meant to fix what is wrong with your back. Its purpose is to help you keep going when you need to, particularly after an injury or when you are dealing with chronic pain.

The available prescriptions now target the symptoms; not the actual problem. If you break your leg, you go to the doctor to have it fixed, not just to get a prescription to deal with the pain. If you have pneumonia, you go to the doctor to get the right mix of medications and recommendations to help you get better – if you have pneumonia, you cannot simply take a drug and get better. You have to rest and convalesce before you can resume your normal routine. And you are going to make sure you are better before you try to go back to your normal life. If you start feeling pains in your chest, you aren't going to take a pain killer and keep going – you are going to head to the hospital or a doctor's office and have it checked out to see if it is heart burn or a heart attack. Back pain may not be as obviously dangerous as pneumonia or a heart attack, and you probably aren't suffering from a pain that is comparable to a broken leg. This is what leads people to overestimate their ability to cope with it, and to try to stop the pain instead of addressing the actual problem.

There are definitely some lifestyle changes you can make that will help you fix the problem, but there are also alternative medications and methods of treatment that can help you heal without relying on opioids or other strong medications.

Looking back on my own personal experience with pain, this is incredibly clear. If I had been prescribed opioid pain killers while in the hospital, I would have been at high risk of addiction because the way the medical profession went about determining the root cause and trying to resolve it was completely wrong. I don't know what would have happened to me if not for my father's friend who was a chiropractor. He was able to determine the root cause and begin the healing process. Sure, there was a lot of pain during that first visit, but it was nothing compared to the perpetual pain I had been in. After that, I just needed to go back for regular visits for therapy. Pain killers were not necessary, and because I was more careful, I didn't continue to exacerbate the problem. When I hurt myself in 2013, it was the same thing, but opioids were an option if I had chosen to go that route. I didn't. Yes, it hurt – a lot. Fortunately, I knew that it was not the right solution for my problem. Instead of relying on medication, I looked for a solution, and that is what got me where I am today. No medication would have been nearly as effective or as fast as the alternative treatment that I received. Not only was the treatment more effective, it was far safer and more natural. This second incident of extreme back pain is what ultimately got me into Regenerative Medicine. It actually targets the problem while helping to reduce the pain; you will probably still need some pain relief through over-the-counter medicines or other types of alternative medicine, but you won't have to rely on them to get you through the day for weeks, months, or years.

    There are definitely times when opioids can be helpful, but generally it is best to use a more natural treatment that works with your body to heal instead of hiding the pain.

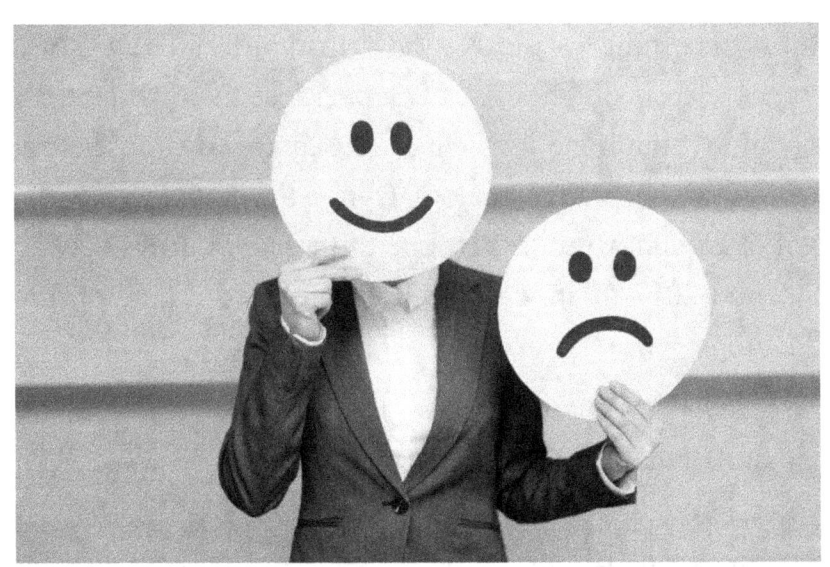

# The Role of Mental Health in Recovery - Angela Smigiel, MSW, LCSW

As a therapist working at The Meadows, a world renowned treatment facility for trauma and addiction in Wickenburg Arizona, I specialize in the treatment of trauma and addiction, putting me on the front line of the opioid crisis every day. Many of the people battling addiction, particularly opioids, were prescribed an addictive medication for a legitimate reason. The problem is that these types of medications are very dangerous and can have devastating effects on a person's life, even when offered for a legitimate reason. With doctors providing refills without even examining patients, there is a very real risk of any potential problems being exacerbated.

According to the National Institute of Drug Abuse, men have seen a higher risk of an overdose than women. The two most common drugs that caused the overdoses were fentanyl and fentanyl analogs (synthetic narcotics), with a total of 28,400 overdoses by one of these two drugs between 1999 and 2017. Pain was the initial cause for many of these addictions.

Over the last decade, I have seen this problem firsthand. I have noticed that many people who are being treated for addiction, anxiety, and depression also suffer from some type of pain, leaving them not only suffering physically, but mentally as they experience withdrawal. Studies have found that people with a significant amount of childhood trauma are more likely to suffer from pain. According to The National Child Traumatic Stress Network, "Throughout a person's lifetime, childhood trauma exposure can be a significant factor in addiction and mental health problems." They estimate that two-thirds of children in the US will suffer from a traumatic event. If not properly treated, these children are at higher risk for underdeveloped coping skills, which increases the odds that they will engage in dangerous and reckless behaviors.

Elizabeth C. Tilson (2018) published the *Adverse Childhood Experiences (ACEs): An Important Element of a Comprehensive Approach to the Opioid Crisis*, examining the correlation between childhood trauma and the current opioid crisis. It should be noted that adults are at an increased risk of addiction if they suffer a traumatic event, but the studies show that those who suffered childhood trauma are at even greater risk compared to adults who typically have a more developed method of coping with trauma and stress.

My work defines ACEs as "traumatic or stressful life events experienced before age 19 and include 8 domains of childhood abuse and household dysfunction, such as physical, sexual, and emotional abuse; adult substance abuse; and household domestic violence." The risks associated with ACEs go beyond just opioid addiction as well, showing that the adults who suffered ACEs are more like to suffer from other issues associated with risky behaviors. Without proper support and a nurturing environment, children are more likely to suffer from toxic stress, which leads to health problems, even if they do not engage in risky behavior as adults. Mental and emotional trauma can manifest as physical pain, creating a psychological cycle that makes them prone to seeking a way of escaping pain. Opioids have proven to be detrimental to people who have experienced ACEs because they are more likely to report pain. They have become much more sensitive to negative sensations, requiring drugs and other methods of escaping the pain.

Anyone who suffers from post-traumatic stress disorder (PTSD) is also at an increased risk of abusing opioids. Since PTSD often goes undiagnosed, it is much more difficult to know when you are prescribing something to a person who has a higher risk of addiction. According to COPE REMs:

- People with PTSD are 50 more likely to develop chronic pain.

- People who have suffered from a traumatic brain injury are 95% more likely to develop some form of chronic pain.

Both PTSD and traumatic brain injury often occur at the same time (such as a concussion from a car accident), which almost guarantees that the patient will be susceptible to addiction, even with monitoring.

An estimated 25 million Americans will be personally affected by PTSD. As many as a third of the veterans who have been on an active deployment are at risk of having one or both of these ailments.

People who suffer from depression, anxiety, or both are also at an increased risk of addiction. Both of these disorders affect how a person physically feels, focusing on the pain to the point where it may feel much worse than it is. Of even more concern is that people who are on opioids are more likely to suffer from depression or anxiety, even if they don't normally have these disorders. Medical experts posit that the relation between a person suffering from depression and chronic pain is that the two problems are linked by a common mechanism. The brain produces chemicals like serotonin and norepinephrine, and these levels shift when a person is depressed or anxious. This changes the way they feel pain, and once their mind latches onto the idea of the pain, it can become almost obsessed with the pain. This does not mean that they are not hurting, but it does increase the likelihood that they will experience chronic pain because of how they perceive pain. As they experience chronic pain, their depression and anxiety are compounded.

It is a vicious cycle that actually pertains to all of these mental conditions and negative experiences.

The mind and body are not two entirely separate entities, as these studies have repeatedly shown. Trauma or stress changes the way a person perceives physical pain. From the chemicals that the brain releases to the perception of pain, people who have suffered from or are suffering from a mental ailment or traumatic event, no matter how far in the past, are much more likely to experience chronic pain. Researchers and medical professionals have found that a person suffering from a major bout of depression is actually more likely to experience chronic pain during the depression,

If you are interested in learning about the connection between mental health, addiction, and chronic pain, *Pain and Disability: Clinical, Behavioral, and Public Policy Perspectives* by the Institute of Medicine (US) Committee on Pain, Disability, and Chronic Illness Behavior is definitely worth reading through for details. It can give you some insights that will help you through rough times or to help know how to help someone you care about.

As a therapist, I practice through a trauma focused lens, so I have seen the reality of the correlation in my own patients. What really informed my reflection on the correlation was the realization that as people addressed their trauma and worked through difficult emotions, often their pain would disappear. My patients often come into treatment after spending years trying to avoid feeling their emotions. I remind them that they cannot selectively numb emotions. As one works to numb pain, shame, and fear through chemical or process addictions, they also numb joy, passion, and love. Initially, I assist the patient in recognizing and connecting to their emotions again. I direct patients to notice where their emotion is stored in their body and then to allow the emotion to surface. Suppressed emotions are stored in the body and begin to wreak havoc. Once patients begin to connect to and feel emotions, I notice tremendous healing begin to occur.

A book that aptly discusses how the body stores trauma is called *The Body Keeps the Score* by Bessel van der Kolk. Van der Kolk puts the universality of trauma into perspective.

> One does not have be a combat soldier, or visit a refugee camp in Syria or the Congo to encounter trauma. Trauma happens to us, our friends, our families, and our neighbors. Research by the Centers for Disease Control and Prevention has shown that one in five Americans was sexually molested as a child; one in four was beaten by a parent to the point of a mark being left on their body; and one in three couples engages in physical violence. A quarter of us grew up with alcoholic relatives, and one out of eight witnessed their mother being beaten or hit.
>
> [...]

It takes tremendous energy to keep functioning while carrying the memory of terror, and the shame of utter weakness and vulnerability.

*Bessel van der Kolk*

What van der Kolk has noticed is that the way the brain perceives pain evolves following trauma, which comes in many different forms. People may associate trauma with a serious accident, a shocking crime, or war, but there are many things around us that can cause trauma. Some events are things that we don't even think about as sources of PTSD because we have, unfortunately, become used to them When the problem is with someone who is a family member or friend, this can make a person uncomfortable with everyone. This undermines not only their ability to trust, but to feel comfortable around others. They are more aware of their surroundings, and their brain is more receptive to negative sensations.

As a trauma therapist, I have seen that trauma can be stored in the body and create an overwhelming sense of fear and pain. This fear, anxiety, and depression carry with them a myriad of chemicals that are associated with pain, such as adrenaline and cortisol. When faced with a trauma, one could go into fight, flight, or freeze response. A person's hormones and the chemicals released by their endocrine system affect how they perceive their world and how they react to it. During the fight or flight response, the sympathetic nervous system stimulates the adrenal glands triggering the release of catecholamines, which include adrenaline and noradrenaline. This results in an increase in heart rate, blood pressure, and breathing rate. After the threat is gone, it takes between 20 to 60 minutes for the body to return to its pre-arousal levels. You can imagine the havoc on the body for someone who is struggling with PTSD and is constantly having the PTSD triggered by their environment.

In the freeze or shut down response the body's systems slow down to conserve energy. The heart rate decreases, the immune response decreases, muscle tone and body temperature decreases, and one may feel hopeless and dissociate from the surroundings.

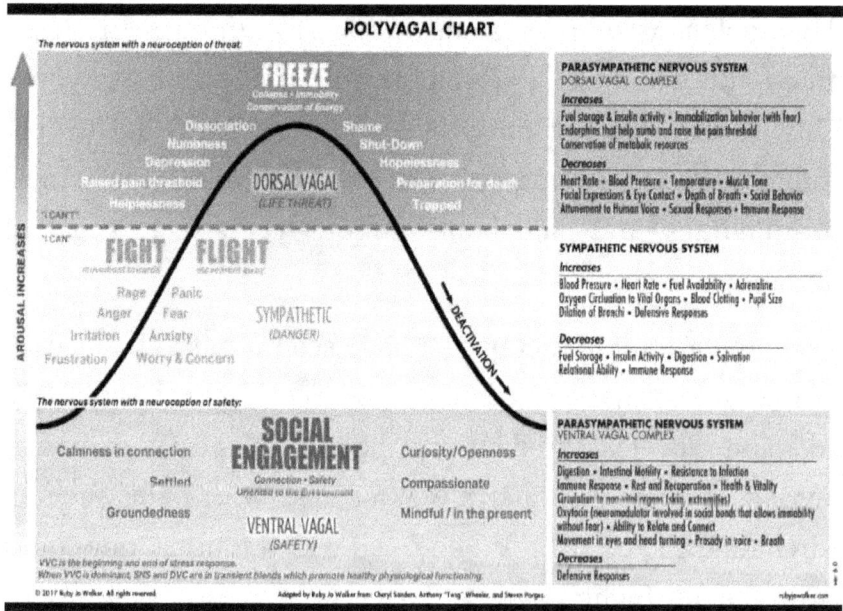

*The Polyvagal Theory*

I have noticed that once a patient has worked through some of their trauma and difficult emotions, their reported levels of anxiety and depression drop along with reported symptoms of pain. When working with a patient individually or in a group setting, a significant amount of my focus is redirecting them to their body and where they notice tension and sensations when processing a difficult event or emotion. The practice of creating awareness between one's emotions and how those emotions effect their body is essential in the healing process. The pain fuels these negative feelings, so that a sufferer is debilitated by the endless pains when they wake. Starting the day like this every day causes further negative emotions, such as stress and resentment. This can lead to anxiety or mood disorders. Unfortunately, the more negative their emotions, the more likely patients are to suffer chronic pain.

## Eye Movement Desensitization and Reprocessing

One of the most effective methods I use when treating patients is eye movement desensitization and reprocessing (EMDR). EMDR works to move maladaptively stored memories that keep a person from recovering mentally following trauma, similar to the way a doctor removes any problems from a wound so that the body can heal. The treatments have eight phases, with the professional assessing the progress of the patient to ensure that it is working.

- **Phase 1:** The therapist talks with the patient to determine their readiness for treatment, and to base the plan on where the patient currently is emotionally and psychologically. The session involves discussing which memories are contributing to the problem, and any current predicament that is enhancing or causing additional stress.

- **Phase 2:** The therapist helps the patient use different ways of handling distress, such as imagery or stress reduction. These are used when the patient feels stressed outside of the session.

- **Phases 3 to 6:** At this point, the patient chooses a target and begins to process it. To do this, the patient needs to do the following during these phases:

- Describe the visual image that relates to the target memory

- Address a negative belief about themselves

- Addres emotions that the memory creates and how it is affecting their physical senstaions

- The patient then needs to address something positive, and compare it to the negative emotions.

- The end of these phases comes when a target memory no longer causes distress because the patient has learned to focus on a positive belief.

- **Phase 7:** The patient begins to focus on closure and keeps a log to see how the positive thinking is helping them to overcome the negative emotions.

- **Phase 8:** The therapist and patient begin to assess the progress.

By 2016, medical experts began to use EMDR to help treat chronic pain. The focus of EMDR is used to help reduce or eliminate the emotional distress following a traumatic event.

Though still in the early phases, studies to date of EMDR therapy shows that patients typically experience different degrees of benefits from the therapy. The therapy treats the emotional and psychological traumas in a way that is comparable to the way doctors and surgeons heal physical trauma. The emotional or psychological block is like a piece of shrapnel that has to be removed before any healing can begin. The focus of EMDR therapy is to help the patient overcome the trauma that has changed the way the patient thinks or stimulates negative emotions.

My experience with this method has been that it is incredibly effective in helping my patients to not only to recover mentally, but to reduce chronic pain. I find this very interesting because it provides one more treatment method that is effective without risking addiction.

## Cognitive Behavioral Therapy

Another method of treating emotional and psychological trauma is cognitive behavioral therapy (CBT). Cognitive distortions or self-defeating thought processes that reinforce the pain can also impede a person from healing from chronic pain. Cognitive distortions include 10 problematic ways of thinking.

1. Patients may see things as being in black and white, failing to understand that there are positives and negatives to everything.
2. They may overgeneralize things, buying into the idea that one negative occurrence is part of a ceaseless negative pattern.
3. They tend to focus on a negative event.
4. Since their focus is on the negative, they fail to recognize or dismiss any positive occurrences.
5. They assume that results will always be negative, ignoring evidence to the contrary.
6. They typically predict that the worst will happen.
7. They constantly magnify the negatives in their life, while minimizing the positives.
8. They tend to cause themselves frequent guilt and shame, usually by focusing on what they *should* have done.
9. Descriptions are usually labeled and described in a way that is creative (and often inaccurate) and triggers emotions.
10. They are more likely to claim to be accountable for something over which they had no control, exacerbating their sense of guilt.

Cognitive distortions causes people to tell themselves, "I cannot tolerate the pain," "I cannot function with pain," and "There is nothing I can do for my pain." These negative beliefs can not only influence the emotions one feels but can also reinforce behaviors and chemical reactions in the body that reinforces the pain.

CBT focuses on changing these constant negative thoughts that feed off each other. It has been documented as a successful treatment method for addictions, anxiety, depression, insomnia, PTSD, and other mental disorders. Since there is a close link between mental disorders and chronic pain (particularly back pain), CBT is regularly recommended as part of the treatment for chronic pain. It is different from EMDR in that it focuses on the present instead of the past. The thoughts that the patients are having now may be a result of a past occurrence, but cognitive distortion can go well beyond just past trauma. Similar to if you begin to limp after an injury, then continue to limp instead of seeking treatment, over time, you will develop other physical problems as a result of the way you adjusted your usual stride. A past traumatic event may trigger negative emotions, but when it causes cognitive distortions, you begin to think in a way that is detrimental to every aspect of your life.

CBT seeks to reprogram the way a patient thinks. There are several types of CBT.

1. Traditional CBT works to retrain the patient to have a positive reaction to pain, such as being rewarded for thinking positively and doing

something about it (instead of focusing on how it hurts, they can't do anything about it, or the pain will never stop).

2. Group CBT forces people suffering from pain and cognitive distortion to interact with other people instead of becoming isolated. Since patients with cognitive distortion tend to drive others away, working with a group gets them to start thinking outside of their heads and pain. The interaction also is likely to decrease anxiety, impulsivity, and depression.

3. Third-Wave CBT uses meditation and mindfulness to get the patient to understand that they can control their thoughts and limit the pain. This is more of a way of disassociating from the pain, but it reduces or eliminates the negative thought process that stems from the pain.

4. Problem-focused CBT focuses on a single problem and targets an outcome. If a patient is suffering from anxiety, the therapist focuses on the thoughts around the patient's anxiety and behaviors to reprogram them.

# The Connection between Mental Health, Chronic Pain, and the Opioid Epidemic

One of the reasons mental health is included in this book is because there are not only many ways to treat chronic pain, but there are many reasons for it. People should use opioids as a last resort and this is one of the reasons why. Any trauma that a person experiences may cause chronic pain, but it is not going to be healed through medication. What is needed is the right treatment, and for mental trauma, that means that the patient needs to seek help in healing their mind to really recover. It is too easy to believe that you don't need to treat your mind if you are feeling physical pain.

If you are experiencing chronic pain and have had a traumatic event in your past, no matter how far back, seeking help for the mental health issue may actually be the best way to not only reduce your pain, but to help you more fully enjoy life. Never dismiss the idea that mental health is not relevant, or think that they are not related. The way that your mind and body work together means that you should never overlook the correlation between mental health and physical health. Treating both can significantly improve your quality of life.

# CHAPTER 7

# Old School versus New School Treatment for Pain

Another issue I have with the way many doctors treat lower back pain and chronic pain is the outdated paradigm they use as a foundation for treating that pain. Relying on pharmaceutical treatments (like steroid injections and opioids) and costly treatments (like 1970's physical therapy rehab and a wealth of different surgeries) does not focus on the root cause. Most of these methods do still have a place – they are all considered obsolete just because they have been around for a while (some of the treatments that I strongly recommend are even older, like acupuncture) – the problem is that they are not as effective at solving what caused the pain. As I've mentioned before, you don't treat the symptom to fix a problem. In the end, you will more likely create other issues, as these methods have proved all too often.

The focus in the new field of treating pain first involves identifying the source of the pain, or what we usually call the pain driver. This is done through a focused analysis of provocative movements that reinforce or release the pain; you need a thorough analysis of the movements that trigger your specific types of pain.

Over time, the focus has shifted from relieving the pain (treating the symptom) to restoring the diseased or injured tissues and correcting the faulty biomechanics or movement patterns that have led to the injury. What I have found during my decades of experience is a problem with the nature of medical schools. Schools today really have not progressed away from the older treatment methods, so the newer methods simply are not being taught in medical schools. Most students leave their long years of studying equipped with outdated methods that mean that they will perpetuate the problems associated with older methods, even when we already know that those methods have limited success and many have far greater unintended consequences. To find the more modern methods of treatment requires a practitioner with a passion for finding real and evolving solutions, someone who is keeping up with all of the advances in pain treatment. It becomes a fine balancing act where the new medical professionals find that they have only reached about half of their goals to be successful at treating pain. As they try to establish themselves in the field, the ones who want to treat the problem find themselves having to continue with their education too. This is a lot to ask of someone who has just finished so many years in school at great expense.

Ultimately, I think that the medical profession is comparable to many technology fields. There is always a better way to do something, so you are in for a lifetime of learning – it really should go without saying. We certainly know better than to try to treat an illness by bleeding someone, the change came about because people continued to study what was best for the body. Newer isn't always better, but traditions don't always hold up. Now that we have a better understanding of the causes of pain, we need to be examining that instead of continuing to focus on simply reducing the pain. And who doesn't like the idea of significantly reducing the pain without the use of medication or the risk of surgery? It's just a matter of getting the field to change the way it is thinking instead of being complacent with the way things are.

# Mechanical Back Pain vs Inflammatory

Back pain may not be a disease, but it is certainly a serious problem. You don't get that many people missing work and major events every year without there being a serious problem. And this is where it really differs from a disease. Diseases are easy to diagnose because we know what causes them; they are typically a result of a virus, bacteria, genetics, or exposure to something dangerous. One of the reasons that so many people suffer from back pain is that it has so many different potential causes, and even different types of pain.

When treating back pain the first thing you have to do is to understand the type of pain a person is suffering from. There are two types of back pain.

- Mechanical back pain is from regular wear and tear that causes a disruption in the way the components of the back fit together. Any repetitive motions that you make or when you overexert your back result in mechanical back pain. Herniated discs, pinched nerves, or strained back are caused by your motions, and they are letting you know that you have been over doing it – that's why your back hurts.

- Inflammatory pain is exacerbated by long periods of rest, with mornings being particularly painful for sufferers. As you start to move around, the pain recedes. Often the cause of this type of pain is related to one of the types of inflammatory spondyloarthropathy, particularly Ankylosing Spondylitis. The pain is a direct result of a degenerative disease and if left untreated can result in the spine becoming fused. With all of the potentially devastating and excruciating problems it can cause, experts like to identify it as early as possible to begin treatment.

My focus is on mechanical back pain since people are the root cause, not a degenerative disease.

# MECHANICAL BACK PAIN

- **Muscle, ligament, tendon strain**
- Discogenic disorders including herniated disc
- Apophyseal joint arthritis
- Spinal stenosis
- Spondylolysis, spondylolisthesis
- Scoliosis

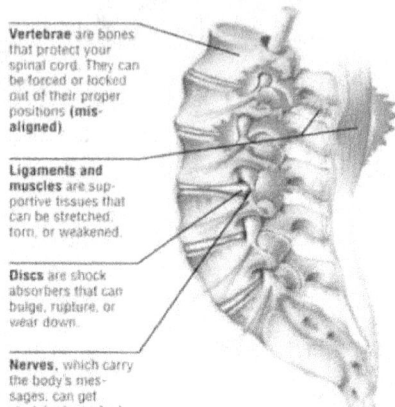

*Things We Do to Our Backs That Come Back to Haunt Us*

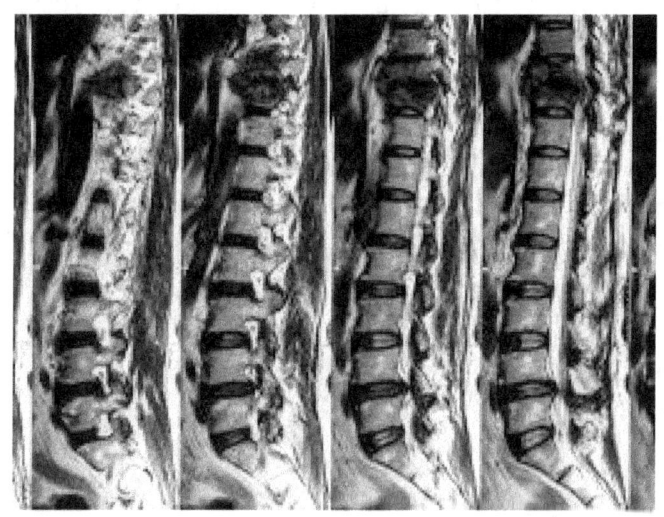

*Scan of an Inflammatory Back Pain Sufferer*

The recommendations I give in this book can be used by people who suffer from inflammatory pain – *everyone* can benefit from this book since we all do things that hurt our backs. However, it is vital to see a doctor to treat the root cause of pain. This book tells you how to take care of your back, both from mechanical back pain and just good practices in general.

Mechanical back pain can be incredibly difficult to treat, which is why so many people rely on the traditional methods, no matter how inadequate they prove to be. To properly treat mechanical back pain, you have to understand the pain driver, and that is something that is far more difficult than simply recommending a couple of over the counter pills several times a day.

# Identifying the Pain Driver

Of course, to understand your back pain and the best way to resolve it, you have to understand what a pain driver is. If you go online and google "back pain driver" what you get is a lot of information about how you can avoid hurting your back when driving, which does nothing to explain what a pain driver is.

A pain driver is the motion or action that you do that causes the pain and it can affect a lot more than just one component of your back. Each time you do a certain action (or more likely a certain set of actions), it hurts the part (or more likely parts) of your back where the wear and tear are. And here is where the problem gets really complicated – it could be more than one action. When you have several different actions that affect multiple components of your back, it can be very difficult to properly identify and treat the cause without creating new problems down the road. Since most doctors learn the traditional methods of treating back pain, they have no idea how to identify and isolate the actual issues.

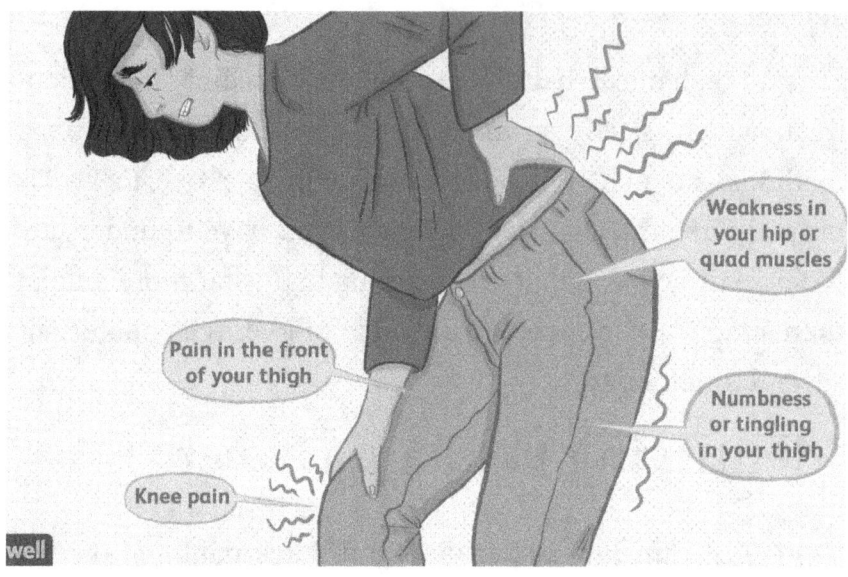

*How Pain from One Component Can Affect Other Back Components.*

When you find a professional who understands that you need more than just a general, unfocused treatment, you can expect that first visit to take you a lot longer it does with other doctors. A proper basic assessment to isolate the cause and affected components takes 30 to 60 minutes. The most thorough exams can take a couple of hours (though very few doctors actually do this since adequate information can be obtained during the basic assessment to start treatment).

This is where my real passion for taking care of people really shows. Essentially, you are looking into all of the little things that people do and figuring out what is actually hurting the back as a result.

For me, this is really the most exciting and enjoyable part of the treatment (well, that and actually seeing people improve, but that is something I enjoy for an entirely different reason). As a child, I used to absolutely love to take things apart and put them back together. Perhaps this comes from my time working in my father's business, but there is something that is just entirely satisfying about taking something apart to better understand how it works. Instead of applying it to boats though, I now apply it to the human body and all of the potential mechanics involved that create a person's pain. There are few experiences that can compare to figuring out what is causing the pain and then helping a person to resolve the issue. The look of happiness when a person is able to reclaim their life without having to do a whole host of little things to minimize the pain is very rewarding.

The human body is just as complex as the most specialized toy, gadget, or device. And the human body does something no machine does – when you hurt, you do things to compensate for that pain. Over time, trying to reduce the pain in one spot without actually treating the pain results in the creation of more pain, just in a slightly different place. Given the length of your spine, there is a lot of room for you to constantly create new pain by failing to identify what part of your back you initially hurt.

By the time people come to see me, they usually have both a primary and a secondary pain driver because they have been trying to remove the pain by changing a motion or habit that they usually do. From holding yourself differently when you bend over, to the way you brush your teeth or put on your pants, to how you walk, there are so many things that we humans do to stop pain, and ultimately we just make more pain for ourselves later.

This is why I constantly tell people not to ignore any pain they have in their back or elsewhere. Trying to compensate for the pain by shifting your body is not a healthy solution to the problem. And it results in two different kinds of drivers.

- A primary driver is the area that is first affected by the regular wear and tear.
- A secondary pain driver is usually results from a chronic pain region.

## Primary Pain Driver

We like to think of ourselves as being sophisticated and knowledgeable, if there is a problem we can identify the source ourselves and act. Admitting that this isn't always true can be difficult in a job or a relationship.

The human body is incredibly complicated. All of those moving parts affect each other, and they can even affect the parts that aren't so mobile. When one part of your body hurts, there are so many possibilities for both what causes the pain and what is actually hurting that finding the source can seem like an impossible task. This is exactly why it takes so long for that initial assessment. Your brain can only tell you that you are hurting – it does not tell you *why* you are hurting. For example, if you have a herniated disc, you may mis-identify the problem as a problem related to an arthritic facet joint simply because the types of pain are so similar and the parts are so close together. Often, it isn't just one part of your back that hurts either, in part because we have a bad tendency to try to stop the pain by doing something that is unnatural to our bodies. For example, a basketball player who has injured a part of his back may find that by walking with his head down, the pain stops. It does not take long for this behavior to become the new norm, but it is doing a lot of damage both around the original pain site and to areas that were not affected before.

Your physician's job is to find out exactly what part of your body is the source of the mechanical pain. This is done through a series of tests that – I have to admit – are going to force you to really feel that pain. This will make it easier to describe exactly what kind of pain you are experiencing, how severe it is, and what motions trigger the pain, or exacerbate the pain. It isn't all pain though. You will also be asked to do actions that reduce or eliminate the pain too. All of this is important for isolating the problem. Inducing the pain and seeing the actions that alleviate pain are all essential to determining what exactly is wrong with your back. It is easy to think that all that is required is to hop into a machine and get a scan, but that really doesn't work. What scans show you is when there is a physical problem. Scans don't show you the cause of the pain if there is no obvious damage to your back.

Secondary Pain Driver

Typically, a secondary pain driver results from a chronic pain region that gives off inflammatory signals, affecting the surrounding tissues. When you take a pain killer, it tends to mute those signals preventing your brain from receiving the signals that are meant to let you know that something is wrong. Clearly, this is not something you should be doing because those signals are the result of your body producing chemicals specifically as a warning. It would be like ignoring an unplanned fire drill. If you were to hear a fire alarm going off, you would not wave it off as an annoyance, pop in some headphones, and crank up the volume so that you couldn't hear the siren. You would look for the nearest exit and leave. Yes, it is a huge inconvenience, but it is definitely better to leave than to stick around and be trapped in a place that is burning. The difference is that it could be a fire drill, but when your body releases pain chemicals, it is always something that you should acknowledge and react to as a warning sign. Your body doesn't produce those chemicals to test how you react – the purpose is always a functional one.

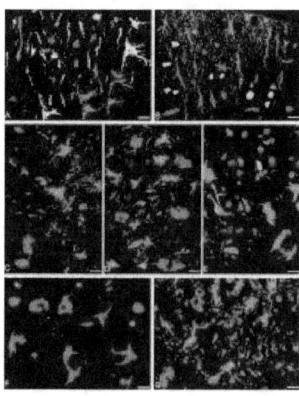

*Image of Chemical Releases*

There are several different types of pain and inflammatory chemicals that your body can produce:

- Substance P
- TRPV-1 and TRPA-1
- $Na_v$1.7, 1.8, and 1.9
- Interleukin-6

It's actually quite astonishing just how quickly your body reacts when you are hurt. Within milliseconds of the pain occurring, your body produces the chemicals, then nociceptros begin to respond to the pathogens and injury to the body part or parts. This is what lets you know that you are hurting, and makes you act to try to remove yourself from a physically painful situation. When it comes to back pain, the way to remove the pain is by adjusting your behavior and physical positioning. This can be a very, *very* short-term fix, but only until your appointment with your doctor. And that should be soon after you start experiencing the pain so that you aren't harming other parts of your back and body.

## Treatment for Drivers

Although they are different, both the primary and secondary pain drivers need to be treated, usually at the same time and on the same day. They are too closely related for medical professionals to treat them as separate problems – they really aren't. Pain has to be addressed in a multi therapeutic approach for the brain and nervous system to develop neural plasticity (how your central nervous system adapts to respond to environmental changes).

Usually, we don't have to spend time assessing the secondary drivers though. Once we determine the primary driver, we can determine the method that will be best to eventually eliminate, or at least significantly reduce, the source of the pain.

# Types of Pain Driver Assessments

We have a number of different types of assessments that help us to identify the source of the pain that go beyond just inducing pain. To understand what is causing and increasing the problems with your back, we have to look beyond just the trigger motions. Both orthopedic and neurological assessments help identify diseased or damaged tissues.

Orthopedic tests are designed to evaluate individuals for musculoskeletal impairment, such as a posture exam and joint stress testing. These types of tests are taught in nearly every medical school because they are incredibly basic and have been established as being a good starting point to determine certain types of problems.

More complex, the purpose of neurological testing assesses a patient's neurological function. This includes several critical aspects of how a person's body functions:

- Muscle strength
- Balance

- How the person's autonomic nerves are functioning
- The patient's ability to feel different sensations

With such a wide range of tests at our fingertips, the initial assessment isn't something that should be rushed through to get a quick fix. Odds are, you will get either the wrong diagnosis or something important could be missed. Since you are likely familiar with many of the types of orthopedic and neurological tests, I'm going to cover some tests that you may know very little about (or you may not have even heard of them since they are not used as often in the medical profession). If you are experiencing back pain, you could actually have this be one of the questions that you ask of potential doctors you are considering, particularly if you look into a specialist to finally treat the root cause of your back pain.

## Functional Blood Lab Analysis

Nearly everyone has heard about blood tests, so you are likely already familiar with the concept of having your blood drawn to have it analyzed for different types of ailments. What most people don't realize is that you can actually have your blood tested to help better understand the types of pain you are experiencing. Yes, blood tests are fantastic for determining what kind of diseases a person may have (many of them typically probably do leave traces of themselves in the blood), but with your body producing chemicals as a warning about the pain you are experiencing, these tests also work to better understand issues about the kind of pain a person is experiencing. The problem is that these tests don't look at everything that could be affecting a patient. If someone goes to the doctor with a host of symptoms and the standard blood test returns with none of the markers indicating that there is anything wrong with the patient, a misdiagnosis is inevitable. By using standard tests that don't look for marks indicated by more specialized tests, doctors and physicians end up treating symptoms instead of the problem. Since they either don't know the problem or have the wrong idea about what is troubling a patient, they will continue to recommend fixes that follow traditional treatments hoping that the treatments will work. Studies have found that the 25 medications that are most often prescribed are for non-specific problems (symptoms, not problems), such as mood, pain, and insomnia. Far too many doctors rely on medications to fix problems because they don't take the time to really delve into the root cause. It's a bit like adding more towels around a dripping sink and hoping that will make the leaking stop. Obviously, it won't.

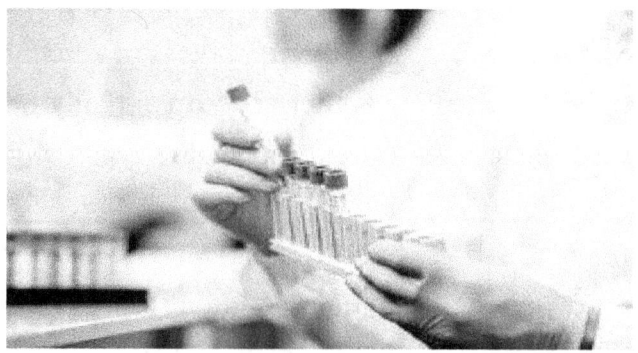

This is where Functional Blood Lab Analysis, also called Functional Blood Chemistry Analysis, can help a physician or specialist better analyze and understand what is going on behind the scenes in a person's body. It can even be used to help prevent serious problems when caught early enough. Instead of looking at the typical blood markers that look for diseases (which completely misses the other markers about a patient's health), it focuses on patients who show a range of symptoms, indicating it is a more complex problem. The tests focus on potential issues that are not yet pathological, meaning the problems haven't manifested themselves, making this a largely preventative means of checking on a person's health. Not all health problems are obvious, presenting themselves in a range of symptoms, as is commonly the case with back pain. It looks at the physiological imbalances to find causes that are more nuanced than the causes of most diseases.

Here are a few of the different types of Functional Blood Lab Analyses that go beyond standard testing.

- Hs-CRP (high-sensitivity C-reactive protein)
- Erythrocyte sedimentation rate (ESR)
- Interleukin 6
- Tumor necrosis factor (TNF)
- A1C
- Triglycerides
- Homocysteine
- Antibodies

Often these tests will help detect other problems, emerging problems, or potential future problems. These tests can also help take a more holistic approach because they don't focus on a problem caused by foreign elements (like bacteria and viruses) or existing problems. They are more comprehensive, and are becoming more common for disease prevention.

## Dynamic Ultrasound Assessment

Ultrasounds are a fantastic tool with applications well beyond the most obvious ones. No longer a type of assessment that is expensive, doctors have begun to look at other potential uses of this incredibly useful tool for understanding pain management (and other applications, but we are going to focus on how to use it to help reduce your pain).

When a doctor conducts a dynamic ultrasound assessment, the images are live, just like with a pregnancy. Instead of focusing on the stomach area though, the patient performs a specific movement at the doctor's direction. As the patient moves, a physician holds the ultrasound probe at the site of interest. This can be multiple places, because as mentioned, everything is connected. By examining the site in question as it moves, the physician can start to see how tissues are functioning. For example if you have a labrum tear in your hip or shoulder, it shows on the dynamic ultrasound image when the tissue gets hung up on another internal structure.

This is very different from the more traditional images because you can actually see the pain triggers as they happen.

These sorts of small signs are not visible to the naked eyes, but the machine provides actual insight into the internal workings of the body.

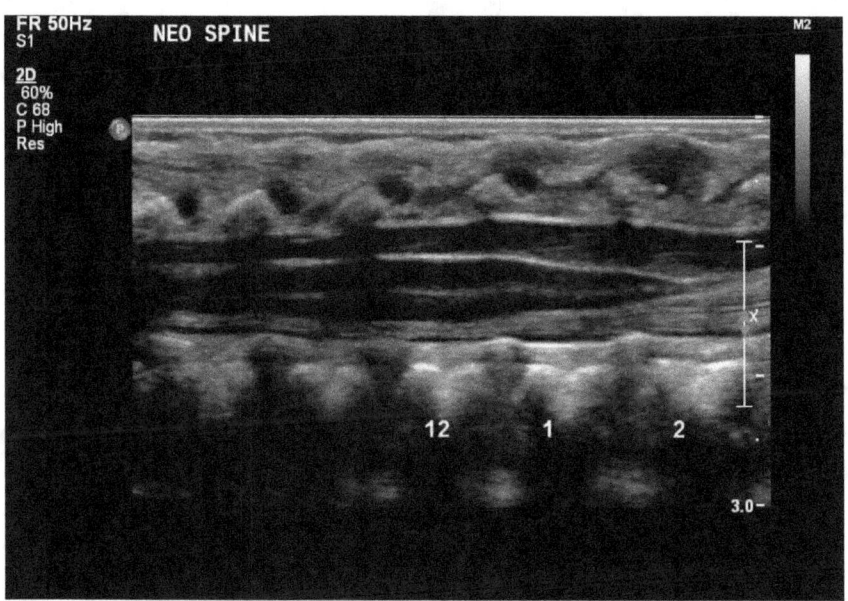

Another benefit to this type of analysis is that it is safe. It isn't producing rays or exposing the patient to something dangerous while allowing the physician to better investigate the problems with the bones, joints, and muscles. The insights that physicians gain through this type of diagnostic look at your body makes the diagnosis more precise. The less guess work your doctor has to do, the quicker you can start getting more meaningful treatments.

Sure, doing the motions that hurt, well, they will hurt. But they will do that anyway. This time the pain will be monitored and better understood. And it isn't just the doctor who can benefit from what the images show. Just like with a pregnancy, as the source of the pain shows up the doctor can start to point out that source. You may not fully understand it, but it can start a dialogue that will help you better understand just what is happening. Once your doctor starts to make recommendations about possible motions that you can do to alleviate the pain, you will understand which parts of the body to engage and which ones you are going to relax.

The more you know and understand about your own body, the more likely it is that you will start to improve the way you treat it. Being more aware of how your movements affect the different parts of your body will help decrease the likelihood that you will create the same problems in the future.

## Gait Analysis

Gait analysis is actually used a lot in sports because the way you move affects how you perform for most types of sports. Some shoe stores use it as well, with the clerks watching how a person walks to recommend different footwear. Some people walk more on the balls of their feet, others put more emphasis on their heels. These are just two things that professionals examine when analyzing a person's gait.

A physician looks at your entire body when you walk to determine how you move and the possible problems your gait is causing. Everything you do affects your back, and your gait is a large piece to the puzzle. Whether you are walking or running, the position that you hold your feet at, the way you move your legs, your stride, how your arms swing, the position of your head – all of it connects to your back. The way your foot hits the ground affects how your spine is compressed. The way you swing your arms reflects in how your back moves exactly opposite to your legs. Like the dynamic ultrasound analysis, watching you in motion helps your physician to better understand how your movements are affecting your back.

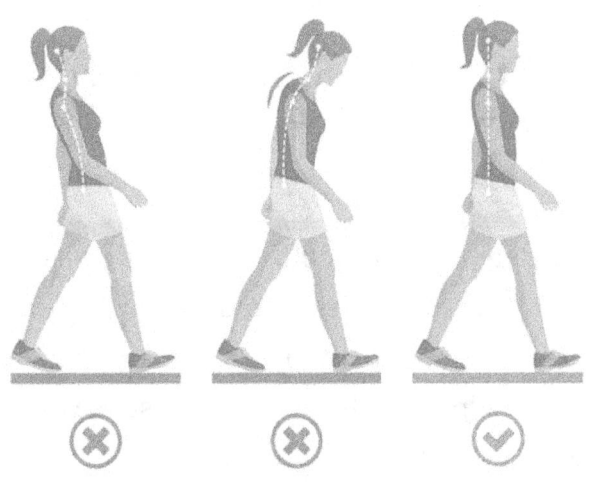

From this analysis, your physician can make recommendations in ways that you can use to start to improve your posture and movements. Yes, it is definitely difficult to make this change because your current gait is so ingrained that you do it without thinking. No one is expecting you to change the way you walk overnight. What your physician wants to see is that you start to be more aware of how you hold your body as you move. When you have been sitting for a while and your back starts to complain, you automatically sit up straight. When you are in motion though, you are preoccupied with other activities, making it less likely that you will pay attention to the same warning signs that make you sit up straight. Also, the constant movement means that the source of discomfort shifts or disappears before returning as you repeat the motion. It is going to take a good bit of dedication on your part to start holding your body in a better position when you are in motion. If you do this at the same time as you try to improve your posture and motions when sitting, you have better chance at success.

# Using the Right Tools to Solve the Problem

There are so many components that we can examine to better understand pain drivers, and there is no one single set of tools to solve a problem. Physicians can use different types of analyses to help solve the problem – just like there is usually more than one way to solve a math problem.

What is key is using the other types of analysis to determine the driver instead of relying on the traditional methods. Technology and a better understanding of the human body have made it possible for us to actually look at the body from a more comprehensive view, instead of making a generic diagnosis and treating a symptom. It can not only help to heal your back faster, it can help you prevent future problems because you are more actively engaged in your back's health.

# CHAPTER 8

## Breaking the Pain Cycle

The problem that you experience with back pain is unique to you because most back pain is the result of accumulated wear and tear. There usually isn't any one thing that is causing your daily pain. For those who do suffer from back pain caused by an injury, there may be some residual pain, but that doesn't mean that you will need to rely on medication for the rest of your life. As the last chapter discussed, there are many things that you can do to manage pain that don't require medication. The mistake most people make is in thinking that they will have to get used to the idea of taking medication or have surgery to be able to resume doing their normal activities, something that simply is not true. Breaking the pain cycle is about a lot more than taking the treatment routes that are most popular at any given time.

This chapter covers the steps you should take to regain control of your life and your pain, and breaking the cycle that is reducing your quality of life. It does mean that not only will you have to be more aware of your habits, but you should start to include some activities that are generally considered enjoyable, such as walking or hiking.

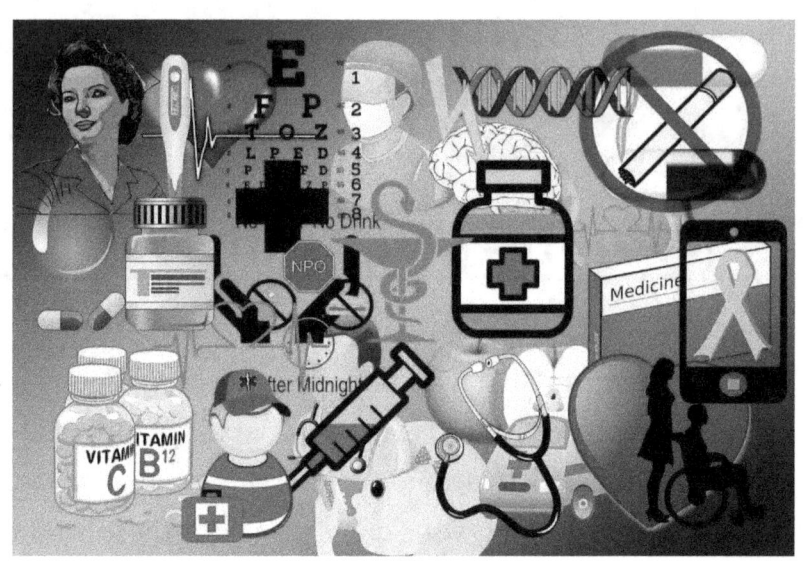

*More Than Just Management*

The thing to keep in mind is that each person is different, so the right solution for you is going to depend on a number of different factors. Find the right solutions for you instead of comparing yourself to what is working for others. What is working for your friends is not necessarily the right solution for you. Pain is an incredibly personal experience, and the way you experience pain is unique to you. From your pain threshold to your pain frequency, there are many things that you have to consider when you try to start breaking the cycle of pain.

Also remember that you should work with your physician to ensure you are not harming yourself before starting any treatments, particularly any exercises. You don't want to exacerbate the problem.

# Understanding the Cause

The first place to start should be obvious, but I am constantly surprised by just how many people are not aware of the motions that cause their pain. For people who were injured, there is at least a starting point for understanding the cause of the pain, but over time you could have contributed to the pain by continuing to make certain motions or doing particular activities.

The best way to start breaking the pain cycle is to get a thorough assessment of your back. It is essential to understand exactly which movements are triggering the pain. As I mentioned in earlier chapters, if you only feel the pain when you lean over as you are brushing your teeth, that is an indication of the motions that are causing you pain. In this instance, the way to eliminate the pain is to simply use a proper hip hinge (a movement pattern). Since brushing your teeth is an action that you do several times a day, every day, you are constantly affecting the area in ways that will perpetuate the pain. A simple change to your routine will not only stop the pain, it will allow your back to heal so that it won't cause you pain in the future.

I am not going to say that a lot of the pain that we feel is caused by improper movements, but a lot of us are guilty of doing things that we know are going to hurt our back. From leaning over at the hips instead of using the knees to pick up a box ("It's so light, this one time isn't going to hurt me") to slouching ("I can't be expected to sit up straight all of the time."), all those little things contribute to weakening our backs. Some of the motions that we do are far riskier than others. If you slouch only occasionally, that almost certainly isn't the reason for the pain. If you bend over the wrong way to pick up a box once, you are almost certain to do it again, and that is going to manifest itself in regular pain.

In my experience, the pain is usually caused by activities that we do every day, like brushing our teeth. The motions are small, but with daily repetition, it is like picking at a scab. Every time you do it, you are just re-injuring yourself.

If you want to break the pain cycle, you have to know the reason for the pain. Your available options are going to change based on the root cause – in some cases you may find that more than one problem is contributing to your pain. You will need to tackle all of the problems that are contributing to the pain. Even more frustrating is when you have multiple pains, with one pain being the root cause for all of the other pains you feel. When you are in pain, you walk a little differently. Two weeks later, you've been compensating for the pain every day, and now you are hurting higher up on your back. Think of your spine as being like Dominoes. When you hurt one part of your back, it isn't surprising when the pain starts to present itself in other areas. We are far more likely to take an over-the-counter medication to get through the pain and then just compensating for the dulled pain by adjusting our posture. You aren't stopping the pain, you are compounding it.

An assessment will help you understand how to deal with pain as you work to treat the real problem. Even if you have injured your back, giving you a good idea of the problem, the assessment can help determine things that you may be doing that could possibly make the situation worse if you keep doing them. Just like a constant, inexplicable pain in your stomach is going to convince you to visit a doctor, you should consider seeing a doctor if your back is hurting. Just because most back pain isn't likely to be lethal doesn't mean that you should feel confident that it will just go away. Pain rarely goes away just because you ignore it. At some point, it will come back, and it will be worse every time it recurs. Knowing the source of that pain is the best way to not only treat the problem but to break the pain cycle.

Even if your back pain is caused by an illness or aging, you can break the pain cycle. It isn't unheard of that the assessment will help uncover other problems, and it could be that you will be told to get other tests to determine if you have a problem. If you already have a known issue, that will affect the solutions that you will consider.

Knowing the cause of the problem is essential to helping you determine what the right path will be for you to break the pain cycle.

# The Difference Between Pain and Damage

When it comes to the back, people tend to confuse pain with damage, which is not true. When you hurt your leg, you don't assume that there is damage to it. The reason that your leg gets better is that you tend to stay off your leg, changing your activities for a while until you think your leg has mended. This is not something that most of us do for our backs.

There are many instances when a person can have a herniated disc and not feel much pain. Some people suffer from chronic pain, but their problem is not going to show up on a scan because the problem isn't caused by damage to the spine. This is exactly why an assessment is necessary, and why relying on medication (or considering surgery) simply is not going to help you.

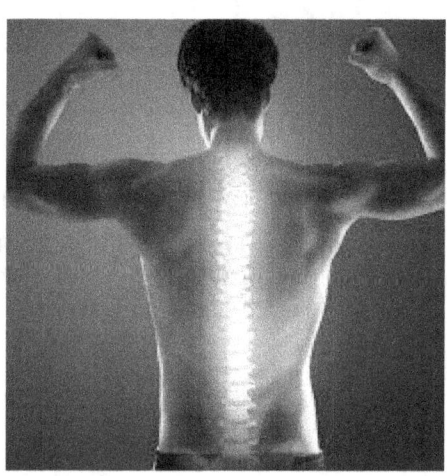

Many people with chronic pain don't have an obvious cause, which can lead to a lot of obvious frustration.

Traditional doctors may tell you that it is all in your head because they can't find an obvious cause. This can result in your doctor prescribing medicine that really isn't going to do what you want it to. Sure, you will be able to do more because the pain is masked, but once the medicine stops working, the pain will return, meaning you will be right back to where you were before you started taking the medication.

We want to be able to trust our doctors, and you should be able to do just that. However, the medical field still has a long way to go in some areas. Most doctors will understandably look for the obvious to treat a problem that is caused by something other than apparent problems. While it may not be a perfect comparison, some back pain has a source that simply isn't observable, just like depression doesn't have an obvious cause. For a long time depression was considered a fake illness because doctors could not see a root cause. Sufferers were told that they just weren't adopting the right perspective or that they needed to toughen up, something that we now know was absolutely detrimental to a sufferer's mental health.

If you are feeling pain in your back, there is a cause, but there are good odds that the cause isn't going to show up in a scan. That doesn't mean that your pain is invalid or isn't real, it just means that you need to seek treatment that does not conform to the "norm" for back pain sufferers. In my opinion, the less traditional methods are far better and should be the first resort and not the last, perhaps because that pain is often caused by something that isn't going to show up in a scan.

Breaking the pain cycle for the less obvious causes of pain means looking at treatments that have proven to work to stop pain, as well as the assessment, to determine the triggers for the pain.

# An Apprehensive Anticipation of Pain

Chronic pain can have lasting effects, moving it from nociceptive pain (pain that is caused by tissue damage) to neuropathic pain (pain that affects the nervous system). This still doesn't mean that the pain is in your mind – it means that your nervous system has been conditioned to anticipate pain. Certain conditions make a person prone to neuropathic pain:

- Obesity or being overweight
- Bad posture
- Brain chemistry that is unique or that predisposes a person to anxiety or depression

If you are constantly expecting to feel pain, it is more likely that your expectations will be fulfilled. Part of dealing with this anticipation of pain, which makes you more aware of little pains you likely wouldn't normally notice, is to start to re-condition your thinking. Activities like functional rehabilitation and meditation can be highly effective because they can help you to focus on something else. Placebo effects may be more effective for these cases as well because the person suffering will start to focus less on the pain they may feel and will start to focus on healing.

## Levels of Pain

Pain is not only a unique experience, it is layered. To break the cycle, you have to address the different layers, particularly for neuropathic pain. Breaking the pain cycle goes beyond just the pain, and often requires you to take steps to change your life. This is much easier to do when you take on your pain on multiple layers instead of just getting treated and resuming your normal routine that will cause the pain to return.

The first place to start is with knowledge. Without knowledge, you are pretty much doomed to have to deal with pain for the rest of your life. You can't break the cycle without understanding all of the different aspects that are causing your pain and what will work best for you as an individual. Understanding is always critical for any problem, even something that seems to be as mindless as back pain. With knowledge, you are much more likely to start making the necessary changes to stop the pain.

Treatments are the next layer, and as the previous chapters have shown, there are many of these. Once you know what is causing the pain, you can seek the right treatment to start to heal that cause. Often the best treatments are going to be regenerative. They may not provide the immediate relief like medication does, but they will start to treat the problem. You can couple the regenerative solutions with medication to make it easier to cope with the pain, but remember to reduce the doses early in the process, even when you use over-the-counter medications. You want to find treatments that stop the pain, and not mask it.

Once you get rid of the pain, you have to ensure that you don't cause the pain to return. I'll go into how to do this a little later in the book, but it is the final layer of breaking the pain cycle. Getting rid of the pain may be the goal, but the ultimate goal is actually to make sure that you don't have to go through it again.

# CHAPTER 9

# Start Healing Your Lower Back Today

Getting in to consult with a doctor is incredibly important if you experience regular back pain, but, as I've been emphasizing, there are a lot of things that you can do to help heal your lower back. Even better, some of these suggestions you can do without spending any money. After all, odds are that at least some (if not all) of your back pain is the result of years of mistreating your back. You may need a little help and occasionally some over-the-counter medicine to help you, but your back is like every other part of your body. If you hurt your leg, you are much more careful, but you don't stop walking. Treat your back the same way – don't stop being active, just be careful and don't do the things that you know you shouldn't do. It is so easy to forget to be careful when your back isn't hurting; being more aware and more cautious will help you not only heal your back, but will help keep your back from suffering similar problems later.

Ultimately, the best way to make your back strong and healthy is to change your habits so that your back can heal. This chapter details the way to heal your back; Chapter 10 details the activities that will help strengthen your back.

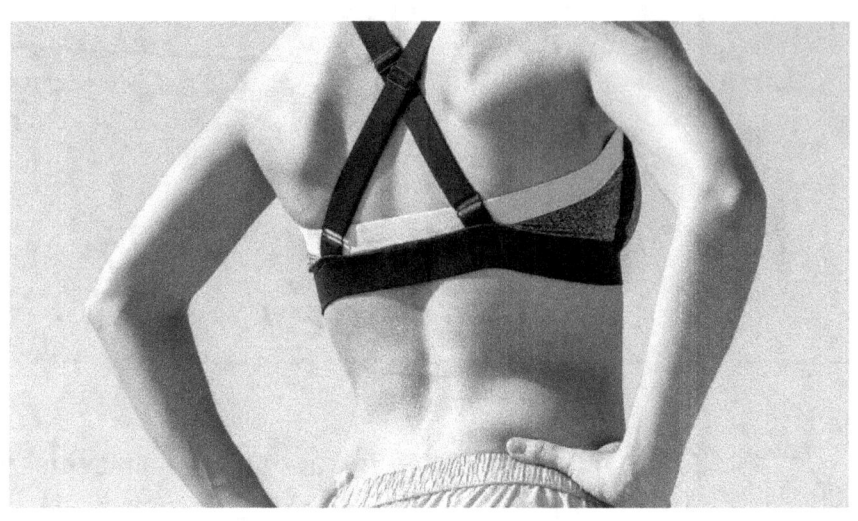

*From Pain to Positive*

Before getting too far into carrying out the ideas recommended in this chapter, consult a physician before you start any new exercise regimen. You have to make sure that any changes to your exercises won't further hurt your back. For most of these exercises, it is best to spend time with a professional who can make sure that your posture and positions are correct. Yoga is a relatively easy way to exercise and has a lot of benefits to both your mind and body, but you can do a lot of damage if you do the poses in the wrong way. This is just one example, but all exercises can potentially do more harm than good when done incorrectly. This is why it is essential that you spend some time with a professional who can ensure you are doing the exercises correctly.

The final thing to remember is that no solution is going to be a quick fix. Healing any part of your body requires a mix of different things, and time is always one of them. Just like what works for other people will have different results for you, and how effective and how long it takes for everyone will vary, too.

## Immediate Action

One of the few benefits of back pain being a nearly universal problem is that we know that there are many things you can do for immediate relief. Many of the treatments that I suggest are probably things that you already know, but some of the things that I suggest may be new or things that you have forgotten. Regarding any of the activities that you do that you know is likely to result in back pain, such as lifting heavy objects or playing a sport, you may want to reduce the time you spend doing them or skip the activities entirely. When you know that you are going to be active, schedule a time to do the treatments too. As you get older, you really have to get accustomed to giving your body the appropriate time to recover – no, it's not great, but it is far better than having a lot of pain and spending several days with significantly diminished abilities.

Don't forget that you can take over-the-counter medicine if the pain is a little too intense and you need to focus so that you can get through your day. Fight the urge to rely on medications, but you can take them on the rare occasions. As you get better at being aware of your posture and habits, your back will stop causing you as much trouble, and you will only rarely feel that these medicines are needed.

## Cold and Hot

The use of cold and hot are classic treatments and they are still quite effective. Both of these treatments are effective during different points in the pain process, and you have to be careful about when you use them because you can actually hurt your back if you apply the wrong solution.

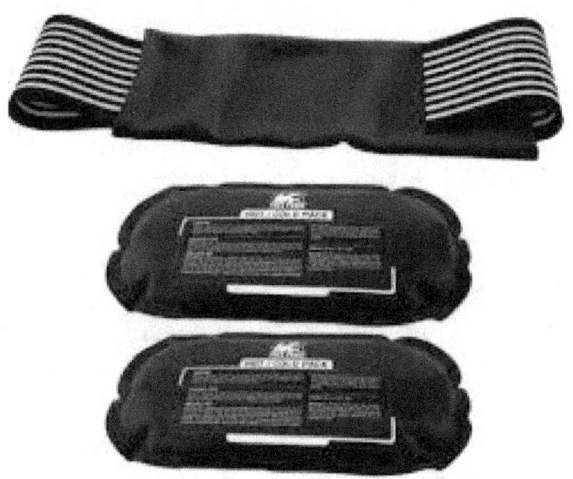

*Ice Packs and Heating Pads – Easy and Effective*

When your lower back begins hurting, apply an ice pack to it. The cold reduces the swelling, which means that your pain will also be reduced. Tweaks to the back are an annoyance, but you don't need to take something over the counter to fix it. Ice packs will give you an immediate distraction because the cold will be very uncomfortable initially. There are cold packs that you can purchase and store in your freezer, but you can also place crushed ice in a hand towel to get the same result. The important thing is to make sure that you don't put the ice pack directly on your skin; it should seem obvious, but if your back is hot, you may think you are alright just putting the ice directly on your skin. Don't. It can hurt your skin to have ice placed directly on it.

Keep the cold pack on your back for 10 minutes, then give your back a break. If you want to apply it again, give your back at least a 10-minute break. You can do this for the first 48 hours, applying an ice pack when your back starts to hurt after you initially start to feel the pain.

It is important not to apply heat during the first 48 hours. Heat releases chemicals that will actually cause greater inflammation. After two days, use the same method of applying heat to the area that you used when applying the ice pack, keeping in mind that you shouldn't keep the heat on the affected area for long. It is very tempting to fall asleep with the heating pad on your back, but that can be very bad for your back. Not only can it burn your skin, but it will raise your blood pressure. Heat may be more comfortable than cold (except in the summer), but you still need to keep its use to 10-minute increments.

## Update Your Work Space

Whether your pain is caused by regular wear and tear or an injury, your workspace needs to be adjusted to encourage a healthy back instead of reinforcing the pain. Your chair is important, but you also need to keep your legs at a healthy angle. Some foot rests can encourage you to keep better posture, and adding a pillow to your chair and placing it in the right place are things you can do to help you reconfigure your sitting position. Your keyboard and mouse also need to be at a comfortable height so that you aren't either being forced to slouch or holding your shoulders too high while you work. Adjust your computer monitor so that top is nearly at eye level so that you aren't angling your head up or down.

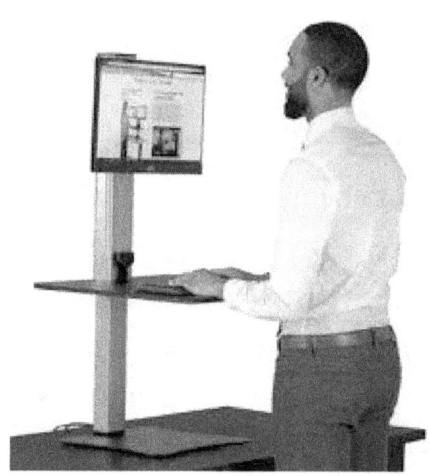

*A Back Healthy Workspace – A Standing Desk Workstation*

A part of the solution is also making sure that you stand up and stretch every hour. Set an alarm on your computer to remind you to stand up every hour. Programs like Outlook make it easy to do this so that your computer doesn't make loud noises that will distract other people. The little pop-up window is fairly unobtrusive, and will remind you just to pop up out of your chair for a couple of minutes and let the load on your back be redistributed. You can use an alarm to remember to periodically stand up, too

Another option is a standing desk. Not all employers are willing to purchase these desks for their employees, but I recommend you see if your employer is willing to make the investment. Standing desks give you a way to stretch your entire body while working..

If you work from home, or if you spend at least an hour at a time at your home computer, then I strongly recommend you get a standing desk. You can buy one that can be placed on your current desk, making it a fairly easy and cheap way of encouraging back health at home.

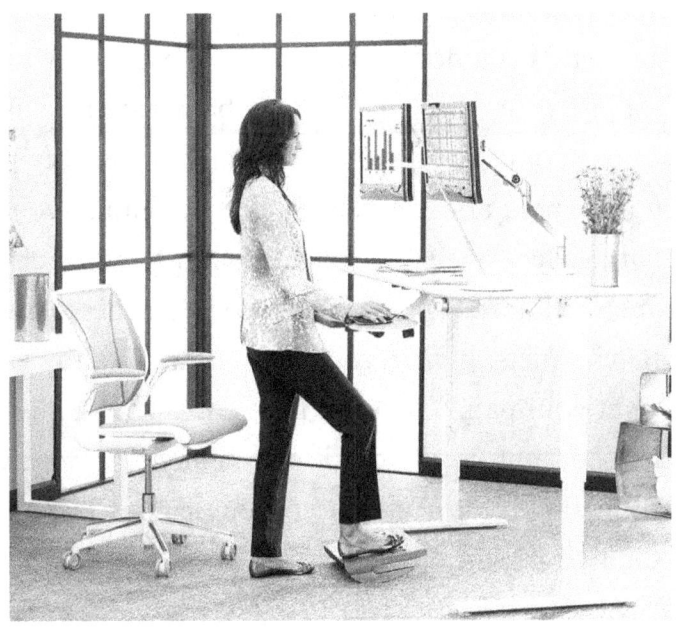

*Standing Desks Provide a Way to Rest Your Back*

Whatever your job, look around your work area and see if there are changes that you can make that will help your back. Whether you are a truck driver or a factory worker there are some small changes that will be extremely beneficial.

# Start Changing Your Diet and Exercise Routine

Depending on the cause of your back problem, you may need to start researching exercise changes and a change in diet. For those of us who spend a lot of time sitting at a desk, both of these are things we know we should be doing anyway, but sitting all day does not encourage better living habits. We eat things we shouldn't – knowing we shouldn't – thinking we can fix it later. If you don't exercise enough or know that you need to adjust your eating habits, that back pain is telling you that later has come and you need to change the way you do things now. There are some diets that encourage you to eat foods that are less likely to cause inflammation, such as the Carnivore, Keto and paleo diets. All of these are anti-inflammatory diets, giving you yet another healthy, natural way to fight your pain. Once the pain ends, you don't have to continue them, but, if you do, it can help you to lose weight while still eating a lot of foods you enjoy This takes care of one of the two important things that people should be doing already.

In the short-term start paying close attention to the activities you do and what you eat helps you start making some of the necessary changes. You don't need to change everything – start taking the steps toward the right habits to improve your life. Again, adopting anti-inflammatory diets can be incredibly beneficial, helping you reduce or even eliminate the pain, but you may not want to continue the diets after the pain ends. Once you are aware of the activities you do all day and what you eat, it will be easier to start making those small adjustments to improve your health. Then you can start modifying your diet to reduce the foods that cause inflammation. You don't need to entirely eliminate them, but making anti-inflammatory food choices the basis for most of your meals will help you in the long run. Making the change to an anti-inflammatory diet all at once is difficult, but if you adjust one meal a day for now, it can help you start to heal a lot faster. Also, follow these diets for your snacks. You will quickly find that you can avoid the foods that are higher in calories or contribute to inflammation.

## Better Sleep

The way you sleep definitely affects your back, and it may be a part of your problem. If you wake up with a sore back (and not because of exercise) or your back feels stiff, you either need a new mattress or you need to find a new position in which to sleep. The latter idea is definitely difficult because you move around in your sleep, but you may be starting in a position that encourages the pain. Putting a pillow between your legs can actually help your back if you like to sleep on your side because it shifts the load. Sleeping with your knees drawn up, kind of like the fetal position, can also help. Firm mattresses are also best to stop lower back pain.

## Look at Your Other Options

Set up an appointment with your physician to discuss your other options. Anything I covered in chapter 7 can provide relief to your back in the long-term. Depending on the root cause of your pain, your options will vary. Your physician may suggest specialists, and you can determine which one you will feel the most comfortable visiting. At this point, you need to start thinking about ways to avoid the pain in the future. Prevention of pain is the best thing you can do to start healing your back.

Part of the visit to the doctor should include a visit to a specialist who can assess your current habits and the source of the pain. Even if your back hurts because of an injury, visiting a specialist for a back analysis can help you learn what to do to reduce the pain. As unpleasant as the pain is, it does have its purposes. First, it is letting you know something is wrong. Second, it gives you a way to find out what you are doing wrong, but you can only do so much. This second purpose is that your specialist can analyze your back and then make suggestions on how you can change your motions to keep from further hurting yourself. Specialists all have their own methods, and the amount of time the analysis will take depends on the individual specialist. With the most in-depth assessments taking hours to perform, you are probably not going to get a full assessment. Make sure to find out what kind of assessment the specialist will perform and an estimate of how long it will take. If you already know what kinds of motions are likely to trigger the pain, make sure to bring that up when you are discussing the assessment. Most professionals will still have you do a few other key motions, but they can focus on the known problems to complete the assessment a bit faster. This does not mean that you should just rush through the motions.

You will still need to move slowly and deliberately during the assessment. First, you don't want to cause further pain or problems by moving quickly; this is more likely to hurt you further than is needed to help the specialist. Second, you will have a better understanding of the pain. Sometimes moving slowly can reduce or enhance the pain, and that is also important to know.

# Planning for the Future

When your back hurts it is incredibly difficult to think in terms of the future. Like trying to make plans when you have a headache, back pain has a way of making it difficult to do virtually anything because of the nagging pain and the fact that everything you do requires the use of your back. What matters is making the pain stop. Once you take a step back and realize that every little thing you do affects your back, it is easier to start taking your health more seriously. From weight loss to more intentional motions to daily activities, there is nothing that you do that does not help or hurt your back. Since most back pain is cumulative, you are going to have to do something that makes all of us groan – yes, even I get annoyed sometimes. Even as I write this book, I am having to constantly correct my posture because after a few minutes, we automatically go back to that usual slouch and rounded shoulders that got us into the trouble we are in now.

Over time, it will get easier, I promise. You are having to undo years of bad habits and ease over your back health. It will take time, which is exactly why this is something you have to plan to do going forward. Reprogramming our brains is not an easy task. Although it may be a lot of work, it is more than worth it. You have had years of knowing that you should sit up straight, lift from your legs, and a host of other things – it was you who chose to do things incorrectly. That back pain is just a reminder that you should be taking the health of your back much more seriously and doing the right thing for your back. If you don't, things can definitely get a whole lot worse.

## Preventative Measures to Keep Your Back Healthy

There are a number of things that you should be doing in the long run, and you already know them. Since nothing in this book is really new, I'm going to give you something more like a checklist because I know that most of us get a sense of accomplishment when we can start ticking things off of a checklist. Planning for the future is never easy. Checklists are just one way to simplify your life and to make regular back health a regular part of your daily routine.

- Regularly assess your workspace for comfort.
- Establish a workout routine that fits your schedule.
- Meditate at least four times a week.

- Visit instructors or therapists who can help you improve your posture and ensure you are exercising properly.

- Do a series of gluteus medias activation exercises once or twice a day to stretch your back.

- Improve your diet, and regularly assess it to make sure you are eating right for your activity levels.

- Establish regular massages or acupuncture to help you relax and do easy back healthy activities.

- Make regular visits to your chiropractor. Chiropractors not only help to realign your back, they can give you tips about your posture and help you determine new exercises to promote a healthy back. If you visit a chiropractor regularly, you are more likely to avoid future back pain.

- Pay attention to your posture, even if it means having a mirror that shows you that sloppy slouching pose you are accustomed to using.

Back health boils down to being more aware of your daily actions and motions. Even if your back is hurting because of an accident, your daily routine is going to contribute to your pain if you don't stay aware of how you treat your back. After having put this stuff off for decades, it's time to start doing what is right for your back. The end results are worth it.

Endorphins – A Natural Pain Reliever

We are too quick to pick up a bottle of pills to ease pain, but triggering your body to release endorphins can be just as effective while actually helping your back heal. They are much better for you in several ways.

- Endorphins are natural, and if you have any kind of "addiciton" it will be to the activities you do to release them.

- Releasing endorphins requires you to do healthier activities, such as aerobic exercise or meditation. That means killing two birds with one stone.

- Massages also help release endorphins. If you cannot be physically active or if you are in worse pain than usual, you can help relieve the pain while relaxing without worrying about movements that will make you worse.

- Endorphins reduce pain while also helping reduce your stress, depression, and anxiety. While pain killers only work on a physical level, endorphins are much more holistic in helping you deal with the pain.

Activities that reduce endorphins are healthy for other reasons, and they will help you long after your back stops hurting. Meditation is actually a great way to release endorphins while helping your mental health and posture. I'll go into how to meditate in the next chapter. For now, just know that meditation and exercise are something you need to start planning to do to heal your back. You already know it, but the endorphins give you a better reason – what is better than a natural pain reliever?

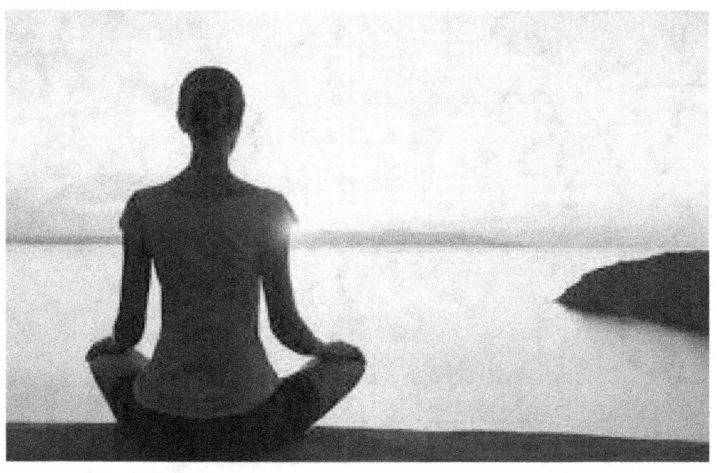

*Meditation for Whole Body Health*

# One Day at a Time

Back pain ranges from a constant, niggling distraction to being debilitating. Regardless of what kind of pain you are experiencing and its cause, it isn't going to go away quickly. Pain is something that we want to eliminate as quickly as possible, and that can make us opt for methods that we would otherwise be inclined to dismiss. In a time of instant gratification, we aren't accustomed to having to put up with anything that is unpleasant (let alone painful) for long. This has been a large contributor to the current Opioid Crisis and is entirely unhealthy for all of us.

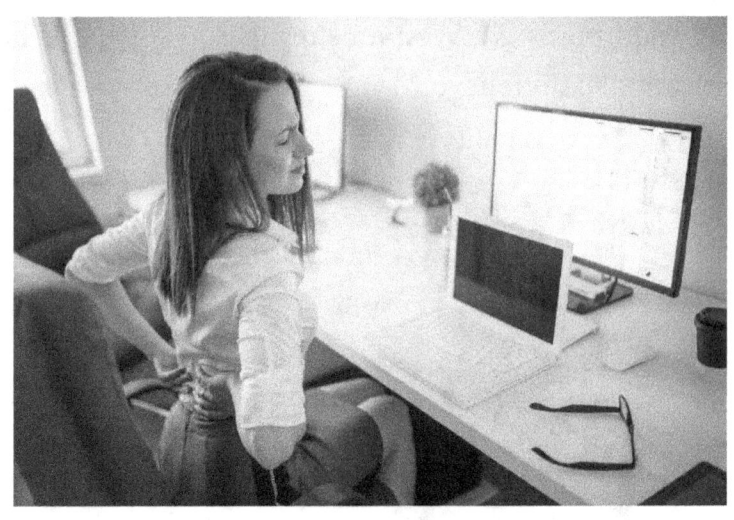

*Working through the Pain*

Healing your back is ultimately about establishing healthy habits that distribute loads across other body parts and relieves stress on the back. Even an activity like sleeping can hurt your back. There definitely isn't much that you can do while you are asleep, but having the right mattress and going to sleep in a healthy position can help.

No one is expecting you to make a slew of changes all at once. Since back health affects literally everything you do, you are going to need to take on just the changes you can manage based on the pain you are already experiencing to determine which changes to make now, and which ones to make later. Some changes, such as changing your workspace, will encourage healthier habits. Others, like exercising and meditation, are going to be harder because you are going to feel as though you don't have enough time. Start slow on exercising and changing your diet to improve the likelihood that you will continue to do them. Very few people are capable of making fast, drastic life changes and being successful. If you aren't accustomed to exercising daily, you are going to need to take it slow. Ditto for eating right. You have to start with an awareness of what you eat. I will help you more with this in the next chapter, but for now just know that all of the changes that you are going to make will help you on a daily basis. After becoming more aware of your habits, it will become a lot easier to start making the right changes. All of those snacks that you eat can be changed to foods that are healthier, and your busy schedule is not going to be quite as packed as you think. Believe me, we all have a bad habit of saying we are too busy, but all you have to do is look at how much time is spent watching Netflix, Hulu, or cable to see that we have time – we are choosing not to exercise. Understanding your daily routine is how you are going to start to heal your back pain one day at a time.

# CHAPTER 10

## You Are in Charge

This could very well be the chapter that you are the most interested in reading, or it is the one that you are going to grudgingly read because you know you should. (If the latter is the case, well done, because I know how hard it can be to force yourself to do something that you really don't have much interest in doing.) I plan to use this chapter to really help you take control over your pain and to give you a starting point for being more pro-active in the health of your back. Back health is absolutely essential to stop being a contributing statistic to the large number of back pain sufferers. It isn't exactly a goal that most people make (most people don't really give their backs that much consideration until their back starts to hurt), but perhaps it should be. If you make proper care for your back a goal, then you are much more likely to be careful of your actions. After all, most of us already know what we need to do to promote healthy backs, but we choose not to do them because they are inconvenient, uncomfortable, or time consuming. Of course, these are just excuses, but after you have experienced back pain, you are going to find those excuses just aren't as good as you once thought they were. If nothing else, back pain has the distinct advantage of making you finally realize that all of those little things that you should be doing are well worth whatever discomfort they may temporarily cause because they save you so much more distress in the long run.

This chapter helps you go beyond just the little things though. From helping you better understand and analyze your habits to correcting certain motions that increase the likelihood that you will hurt your back to exercises that help strengthen your back and core, this chapter has a lot of information about activities that actively help you avoid further pain. I'm not saying that you should try to do all of them at once, but there are portions from each of the following sections that you can start doing today to encourage yourself to keep doing what is right for your back.

Before going any further, I feel it necessary to remind you that you need to talk to your physician about changing your exercises and diet, particularly if you are struggling with your weight or are not accustomed to exercising. For many of the exercises, you should really check into taking a class so that you can ensure your posture and motions are correct.

This is particularly true if you are competitive. What someone else is doing has no bearing on your own ability. Yes, I've seen people in their golden years doing perfect exercises, and it has made me feel like I should be capable of doing more. Then I remembered that people who are doing these kinds of activities well into their golden years have probably always taken good care of their backs. I have seriously injured mine twice. It isn't a matter of age – it's a matter of your skill level and physical abilities. You are doing these activities to promote back health, and that means what everyone else is doing is irrelevant. And yes, I am going to remind you of this again later in this chapter. It is absolutely one of the most important things to keep in mind, and you will need to remind yourself as often as it takes to quit pushing yourself, too.

## Journals That May Help

I may be placing a huge emphasis on exercise (as could be expected), but there are several other things you can do to take control of your pain – and journals are a great start. There are three types of journals I recommend:

- Pain journal
- Diet journal
- Exercise journal

Each of these journals will help you better assess your habits and the pain you experience. They can be written or you can keep them electronically, whatever is easiest for you.

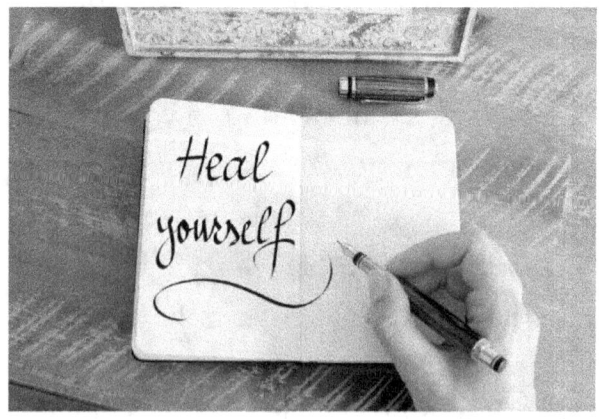

*Journaling to Define and Manage Your Pain*

## Pain Journal

A pain journal may be the easiest journal to keep as the goal is to stop having pain (the diet and exercise journals are probably things you should update at least monthly, even after establishing a routine). You will need to add to the pain journal every time you experience pain and for a week or two after the pain has stopped.

The goal of the pain journal is to understand the source of the pain, the activities that start or exacerbate it, and the duration of the pain. Even chronic sufferers find that they have some days that are relatively pain free. There are hints of why your pain starts while you are going about your daily habits and activities. Every day that you have pain, you should be entering information into your journal about what remedies you took, the severity of the pain, and any motions that changed the pain level (lessening it or worsening it). Then, when you visit your doctor, you can quickly remember all of the details to find a better solution.

Do keep entering information even after the pain has stopped. It could be that something else you do will trigger the pain, in which case you want to be able to look over the journal to figure out what it could have been.

Just a few sentences each day will generally be enough. This will allow you to quickly get through all of your entries. This will also make it easier to start analyzing the other parts of your life that you need to change to promote a healthier back.

## Diet Journal

This journal is the one most people are loath to keep because it shows you just how unhealthy your eating habits have been. It is easy to tell yourself you don't eat so bad until you have a journal staring you in the face and showing you just how unhealthy you have been. Believe me, I know just how difficult it can be to keep these notes. Consider it a necessary evil. I recommend a low carb, non-inflammatory diet such as carnivore, paleo, or ketogenic for my patients.

The best part is, you don't have write down everything you eat. Just snap a picture, and store that in a digital journal to show what you have eaten over the course of the day. There are also a lot of free apps that can encourage you to be more aware of the calories and make recommendations for better snacks. Since this is easily the hardest of the three journals to keep, whatever you can do to make it less of a chore will make it easier for you to start tracking your diet so that you can improve it. See where you can start adapting an anti-inflammatory diet into your current eating habits. Making such a large change all at once usually doesn't work, but if you start to change your snacks and one meal to something like the keto diet, you will have an easier time of transitioning your entire diet to something healthier.

## Exercise Journal

An exercise journal may seem rough at first, but it is the one that can easily make you feel the most accomplished in about a week. Whether or not your back feels sore, the fact that you have increased the amount of exercise you do over the course of a week can be absolutely exhilarating. First, you may start to feel a little healthier – even if it is more of a placebo affect (one week of exercise does not undo years or decades of too little exercise), it will encourage you to keep going. Use that boost in confidence and feeling of accomplishment to keep doing it.

I recommend avoiding the scale for a bit when you start exercising. Yes, you do need to know your weight, but for a little bit, avoiding the scale can actually help you keep on track. In most cases, you are either going to have the same weight or you will gain weight. Neither of these is encouraging when you are trying to establish and maintain a regular exercise schedule. Just avoid the scale, and let the sense of accomplishment for finally starting the journey to getting healthier be the reward you need.

Aerobic exercise should be included in your routine, even if it is just walking more daily. I cannot emphasis enough just how important it is for your back for you to be in motion on your feet. Experts recommend at least 20 minutes of sustained walking a day, but I recommend going for at least two 20-minute walks (or 1 jog and 1 walk) a day. I know that for most people, if they aren't exercising, then they are sitting down. The more walking you can work into your day, the better it is for your back.

# Correct Motions to Reduce Stress and Loads to Your Back

One of the hardest things to do to support your back is to change the way you have been doing things for years (or decades). Just like you should be more aware of how you sit, you should pay more attention to how you move. Everything you do can potentially be a trigger for back pain. Leaning over the sink while brushing your teeth, putting on pants, even opening doors can hurt you if you twist or stretch your back incorrectly. It is so easy to do something wrong once or twice, and then have that become a very unhealthy habit. Yes, it seems like it is too easy to say but, honestly, it's the little things that we do every day that really cause our backs the most problems. It's kind of like brushing your tire against the curb pulling out of the driveway or away from the side of the road. Doing it a couple of times won't affect the tire much, but when you do it every day, it wears down that tire much faster.

It is definitely important to brace yourself and engage your core when you lift, but ultimately, you should always keep your core engaged. When you walk or jog, most people tend to engage their stomach muscles. However, most of us don't engage them when we are sitting or standing. We let go of our stomach muscles, putting all of the work on our backs. It isn't easy, but the better your posture when sitting or standing, the more likely you will be to keep your core engaged.

## Hip Hinge

As promised, I want to take a bit of time to talk about the hip hinge. This motion is easily one of the best ways to promote a healthier back, although it will admittedly probably take a while for you to start doing it properly. Just try to be more aware, and over time it will become almost second nature. If you don't adjust any other motions (although you definitely should), make sure you start being more aware of how you bend over.

The way that most people bend over is to lift their torso and stick out their necks, meaning they are using their upper backs to do most of the work. The hip hinge uses the ball and socket part of your hips (which were actually designed for bending over) and your glutes (since they are the biggest muscle in the body, you should be putting them to more use). This takes the strain off of your spine, which was not designed to be used a lot when bending.

I can describe how to do a proper hip hinge, but reading about how to do it adds unnecessary risks. Instead, take a few moments right now to go online and watch a short video on how to do it. There are so many videos that show this movement that you would be much better served in using the video over trying to interpret text. The visual alone is worth a lot more than words to make sure you do it right. Do make sure to use reputable sources so that you know the method is coming from an expert. You can also watch several videos to make sure you watch the movement from several different angles for the motion, as well as making sure all of the videos are consistent in their method.

The following are some exercises that can help you become more accustomed to using the hip hinge because they force you to think about what you are doing for the full exercise:

- Wall touch or wall slide
- Kneeling squat
- Banded hip hinge

This does go beyond just bending over to pick things up though. If you don't use a hip hinge for all of your forward movements, including leaning over when you brush your teeth, you are going to be putting an undue burden on your back. Try to incorporate the proper hip hinge into everything you do.

## Lifting

This is another action that we do that we tend to do incorrectly. With most of us knowingly doing it wrong, that makes it that much worse. As soon as it becomes a habit to pick up anything the wrong way, you are going to do it again, even for the times when you definitely need to use your legs instead of your back. The reason this is listed second (instead of first is because you can do a lot more harm a lot faster by doing it wrong) is because learning to do a proper hip hinge will help you to remember to lift from your legs instead of your back. Once you have the hip hinge down, lifting from your legs will be a lot easier to do.

Lifting from your legs means involving both your knees and your hips in the process of lifting. Too often, I've seen people lean over to pick up a small box using just their backs (their hips are only minimally involved). It doesn't matter how light the item is, you should always use your legs and glutes to lift. When you don't, you are reinforcing bad habits that you will likely continue to use for heavier items. This is exactly what causes millions of people to have back pain every year.

Just like with the hip hinge, check out proper lifting motions. There are even more videos and illustrations of the proper way to lift objects because companies often have to provide training on this (that is how prolific bad habits have become when lifting).

The trickiest part of lifting is making sure that you always keep your core engaged. If you don't engage your stomach muscles, you are putting a lot of unnecessary stress on your back. It is not enough to simply use your legs (although this is almost always the first mistake that people make when it comes to lifting). You have to activate the lumbar stabilizers to evenly distribute the load across your body instead of putting the full load on your back, or your back and legs.

## Getting Dressed

Compared to the other two actions, this activity can seem entirely silly. However, knowing someone who literally hurt his back while putting on his pants, I feel it is a good reminder that every little thing you do can have consequences on your back. It is actually recommended that you sit down to put on pants or shorts instead of putting one leg at a time through the pants' leg. Sure, this could seem a little strange, at first, but think about how you put your pants on. There are movies where characters jump around on one leg, leaning over trying to get one of their legs into the pants. Naturally, this is an exaggeration, but there is a grain of truth to it. When you dress, you are twisting your back when you put on pants one leg at a time. No, it may not be much, but over a couple of decades, that "not much" can amount to a lot of wear and tear on your back. Instead of risking the little pains, just sit down and slip both legs into the pants, shorts, skirt, or dress. You may even find that you save just a little bit of time because you can avoid having to wiggle both sides before slipping the clothing over your hips.

I would recommend applying this to your shirts as well, though you are far less likely to hurt your back from improper twisting. Button downs are more easy to put on when you use both arms at once than if you slip the shirt on one arm at a time anyway.

## Gait Analysis

You can start your own analysis of your habits as you wait for your scheduled appointment with your physician or a specialist. When people are in motion, they are typically at their best. Your core is engaged, you probably stand a good bit straighter, and your weight is distributed more evenly because you are moving. The way you walk is called your gait, and it can play a role in back pain. If you slouch when you walk, that can harm your lower back. If you favor one leg over the other, that can hurt your back (and at least one half of your body as it was not designed for you to place more weight on one side over the other). Exaggerated movements when you walk can also do some damage.

When people experience lower back pain, they are more likely to modify their gait, at least for a while, to compensate for the pain. If you are sick or injured, that can also result in a modified gait.

The full gait cycle begins when your foot touches the floor as you walk. You then begin to shift your weight from one leg to the other. As you shift your center of gravity over to the next foot, you prepare to remove your other foot up off the ground. The cycle ends as you lift your other foot from the ground and begin what is called the terminal swing, passing the foot through your center of gravity and planting it on the ground in front of you. About 40% of each step has one of your feet in the air as it goes from being behind you to being in front of you. This is why the way your walk is so critical; 60% of your walk puts all of your weight on one half of your body and keeps you stabilized while you put one foot in front of the other.

Your doctor will almost certainly analyze your gait to determine certain aspects of the source of your pain because your gait reflects any compensation you are doing to prevent pain. That doesn't mean you can get a rough idea about your own pain. The following are some of the most common types of gaits associated with pain.

- An antalgic gait is usually refered to as a limp. You are more likely to limp for pain in your knee, ankle, or hip.

- An ataxic gait is an uncoordinated or unsteady gait. An exaggerated type that isn't related to pain is the way someone who has imbibed too much walks. It is most often seen in people who suffer from a cerebellar ailment.

- People with Parkinson's disease or other similar diseases often exibit a festinating gait. Each individual step is usually shorter and taken more quickly.

- The high stepping gait is often used by people suffering from a weak anterior tibialis. Their feet tend to drop, so they over compensate by lifting their feet higher to keep their toes from draging.

- If you have weaker hips or gluteal muscles, you are more likely to have a trendelenburg gain. This is similar to a waddle as you lean a little to the side as you walk.

There are a number of other gaits that you can check out at www.thegaitguys.com. They can give you a better idea of what your particular gait means, whether you are in pain or not. If you are walking differently to alleviate your pain, you are going to need to focus on how you walk as your pain subsides. You may also find it incredibly beneficial to adjust your usual gait to more evenly distribute your weight as you move. Of course, holding your shoulders back to help keep your back straight – and not walking with a cellphone in your hands – will help you take better care of your back.

There is also a video called Gait Analysis that will help you to determine which muscle or muscles need to be rehabilitated - https://www.verywellhealth.com/gait-meaning-and-cycles-2696126.

# Exercises to Help You Be Kinder to Your Back

This section is dedicated to the actual exercises that can really help your back, so long as you do them in the right way. Before jumping into the exercises though, I want to give you a few reminders and a warning.

Learning how to do these stretches, and exercises right is necessary to help instead of hurt your back. Don't rush through the poses either. Poses and motions can do as much harm as good when they are not executed properly.

When you do each exercise, focus on the pose or motion. Here are a couple of things to keep in mind when you get started.

- f you have issues with your balance, use something to support yourself. Even if you have exceptional balance, strengthening your core often means relearning how to stand and move. Use equipment, blocks, walls, bolsters, or some other sturdy object when you need to.

- Remember about the proper hip hinge and use it. If you have lower back problems, forcing a motion or exercise is going to trigger or exacerbate them.

- Always start a new exercise, regimen, or fitness program with an instructor. If you are already a back pain sufferer, you need the help of a professional for at least a few months to ensure you do the movements correctly the first time, and then that you don't get sloppy as you get more accustomed to doing the exercises.

Before you do any exercises, you need to make sure that you are engaging your core. You have to develop your abs so that they will offer enough support to do the exercises. They will stabilize your spine. The exercise routine that you choose needs to take your current abdominal strength in mind, and you will need to make sure to keep your mind on keeping your abs engaged, as well is on keeping your movements controlled.

## Gluteus Medias Activation

This one isn't really an exercise so much as a set of exercises that will help you strengthen the area that can really help provide your back with more support. It doesn't hurt that this set of exercises can also help shape that area, making it look firmer and more appealing. That is definitely a side benefit though, because the primary purpose of these exercises is to strengthen your hip muscles. After sitting all day, engaging them will help undo some of the damage while making them stronger – which ultimately means you are more likely to do other things right, like the hip hinge and the way you lift objects.

The following exercises are great for strengthening your gluteus medias:

- Horizontal leg lifts
- Isometric wall lean
- Clamshell

There are a number of exercises that require the use of a rubber band and can really help you activate these muscles, but you definitely need to have a trainer help you with doing those properly. A trainer can not only make sure you are doing it right (from the way you wear the band to the proper movements to fight the resistance), he/she can recommend the best ones based on personal experience.

## Piriformis Stretch

The name of this exercise refers to the muscle you are working. The muscle isn't big, but it can really help you when it comes to taking care of your back. For those of us who spend a lot of time sitting, taking the time to use this muscle will really help you feel less stiff. It is another movement that you do while lying on the floor, giving you more time to feel a bit relaxed while targeting a difficult muscle to work out.

## Core Stability – Pelvic Tilt

The primary purpose of this exercise is to help build your core. With stronger abs, you will not only give your back a lot of support, but you will start to feel better about yourself. It is another exercise you do while on the ground, but you start by engaging your stomach muscles. As you do this stretch, do make sure to follow these rules:

- Your feet should always be flat on the floor.
- Make sure that your shoulders are always pressed into the floor, but you should not be straining to do this.
- Make sure you keep breathing – yes, this seems like a given, but when engaging their stomach muscles, people do tend to hold their breath.

## Pelvic Tilt

This motion is a lot like yoga's bridge pose, but your shoulders don't leave the floor, and you continue to move your pelvis instead of holding it in place. This exercise can actually help to relax your upper body while working your lower body, but you do need to be careful not to move too quickly just because it is easy. Make sure you keep your stomach muscles and gluts engaged, otherwise you will be forcing your back to do even more work.

## The Bird Dog

You start this pose on your hands and knees, which may make you feel more comfortable and less cautious about your movements. During the entire exercise, you will keep your core engaged as you move one arm and one leg. You will need to be careful that you don't allow your back to sway as you move.

This is one of the more advanced exercises, so you need to make sure to do this one with a trainer or expert to ensure you aren't doing it wrong. It seems like it would be an easy enough exercise, but if you do it wrong, you can hurt your back. Rely on your chosen professional for a while to ensure you have the motion down before you try to do it on your own.

## Meditation

Technically, this isn't physical exercise, but it definitely has physical benefits. Meditation requires you to hold a straight-backed posture for the duration of the exercise while you clear your mind and basically give it a reboot. The whole point of this exercise is to force you to stop and to give your mind and body a break from the constant demands you make on them all day. You can start your day with meditation, end the day with it, meditate in the middle of the day, or bookend your day with it (which I recommend, especially when you first start trying to change your habits).

As you meditate, you should keep your back straight. Since you aren't supposed to be thinking about anything else, your mind should be forced into the moment when all that matters is your breathing and posture. Nor do you have to do it for a particularly long time. A couple of minutes is enough if you are busy. It is best if you can meditate for 10 to 15 minutes, but this can be very difficult in the beginning since most of us aren't able to sit still that long and not try to get a million other things finished. It may look like you aren't being productive, but after you have become accustomed to meditating, it is very difficult to stop. It can help you feel a sense of calm that is not possible otherwise. Like a good exercise session, meditation can help you feel a lot better. And you don't have to worry about being sore when you are finished. If nothing else, it can help you get accustomed to sitting up straight and being more aware of your body, which will go a long way in helping you change your habits in ways that will be better for your body.

## Establishing a Routine

Everyone's schedule is different, and what works for someone else's schedule may not work for you. Since you will need to use a trainer or instructor when you do these exercises, you will need to make sure that you will continue to go to the classes for instructions for at least a few months. You should know that you have the motions memorized before you start to do them when you are alone. If the instructor doesn't have a mirror for you to see how your body should move, ask if you can do your exercises in front of one. At some point, you will want to be able to do your workout without having to leave your home (freeing up your time and money, while keeping you from sitting in the car for one more trip).

When you do start to workout alone, make sure that you have a mirror so that you can verify you are doing the motions correctly. This is why it is important to do the exercises with a trainer and in front of a mirror in the beginning. You should be studying yourself as you move to ensure you are doing the exercises correctly.

You should be challenging yourself, but not to the point that you end up discouraging yourself, and certainly not to the point where you do yourself more harm than good. If you find that your back hurts after a particular day of more grueling exercise, reduce your reps or exercises. Let your back dictate what you do because you are trying to treat it better. That doesn't mean to use it as an excuse not to exercise at all. It does mean that you should listen to your back, so if it is hurting, you need to figure out the cause before doing exercises that could compromise it further.

There will be times when you will be too busy to do a full routine. This is when you need to have an abbreviated workout. There is always time for you to do at least half a dozen exercises for your back because they really don't take that long. If you have time to watch TV, play video games, or sit and drink a beer, you have time to finish a few exercises. In the end, if you make it a priority, your back will heal much faster than if you leave it up to whether you "have time" or not.

If you are the kind of person who tends to stop exercising when you don't have help, then find a support group to help you find your motivation, even when you want to believe you are too busy. Most people are able to keep going when they have people who can act as cheerleaders to keep your motivation up. One great place to start is Open Sky Fitness (openskyfitness.com). It is an app that helps you meet up with other people to exercise, understand functional movements, and becoming a part of the community can give you the support you need to keep improving the way you support and care for your back.

## Physical Therapy

The best way to start to really heal your back and to make the changes more permanent is to seek the help of a physical therapist. Their focus is on helping you learn how to improve your motions and to induce neuroplasticity. Neuroplasticity is the natural progress of your brain to change over time. Habits are formed through neuroplasticity, and this is where your therapist is going to work with you to undo bad habits and start implementing back healthy habits. This could include your walk, the way you sit down, the way you remain sitting (you will get more than someone just nagging you to "sit up straight"), the way you lift, and the way you move. They focus on short-term, medium-term, and long-term changes that will help you treat your back with the care needed to prevent further problems.

More than 40% of chronic lower back pain is caused by lumbar discs. The discs are instrumental for everything you do, so it is not a surprise that chronic pain is often caused by issues with your discs. The combined motions of flexion and compression are the quickest way to injure your discs, and that will cause you a lot more pain than many other types of back injuries. You do this when you fail to use a proper hip hinge or when you lift from your back. Genetics certainly have a role in how much your back can endure before the discs start to exhibit problems, but problems are inevitable if these are regular habits. Nobody has a back that can endure this kind of constant improper use, placing so much stress on your back while leaving your other muscles largely unused.

When your back reaches its tolerance for abuse, you will begin to injure your discs. You may not feel the pain immediately because the inner layers of your discs do not have the necessary neurons to feel pain. That will happen as your discs begin to get compressed. By the time you feel the pain, you have already done substantial damage to your disc or discs.

Physical therapists will help reprogram your physical habits. Trying to do it alone usually does not work. Often people do not realize just what they are doing wrong in the first place. Or even if they do know, they may choose a different motion that does just as much damage or worse.

Your physical therapist will show you how to do the motions correctly, both when you hurt and when you don't.

# CHAPTER 11

## Other Joints

One of the reasons I am such a huge proponent of more natural remedies and improving your habits over taking medication for pain is that by doing more to support your back, you will improve your other joints as well. Any kind of drug you take is going to have adverse effects on other parts of your body and mind. A healthier life style will positively affect your body.

If you are experiencing pain in your back, it is quite likely that you are also managing pain in other joints. By doing more to take care of your back, you are going to do a lot to help virtually every other part of your body. You know that your body requires a certain amount of exercise, so if your body is hurting (not just your back) then exercise based on your current abilities is the best way to start healing your entire body. When it comes to eating right, most of us have a tendency to postpone doing the right thing until the damage becomes obvious. Gaining weight is inevitable for most of us as we age because our metabolism slows down. This is why it is so very important to start eating a healthy diet when we are still young. Still, it is better late than never, and helping your back is just one of the many benefits. Regular exercise and a better diet not only take stress off of your back, they relieve your hips, knees, and other joints.

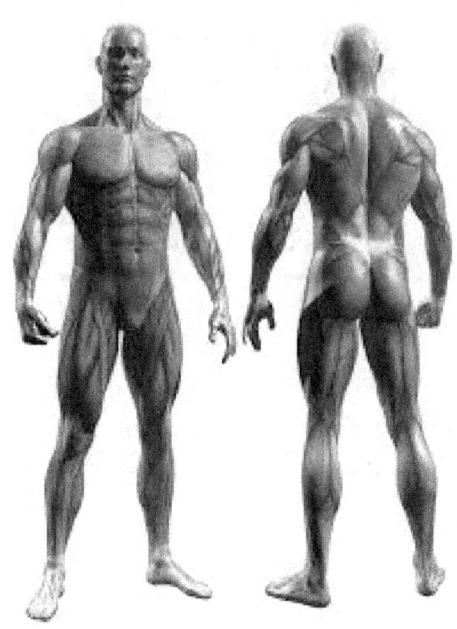

*A Whole-Body Approach to Healing*

Another reason back health is so important is that we have a tendency to change our posture, gait, or other motions to compensate for pain. If you are experiencing lower back pain on one side, you may lean a little more to the other side when you stand or walk. This puts more of the load on that hip and leg, which can do a lot of damage even in the near term. Improperly carrying something like a bookbag hurts that entire side of your body, from your neck to your feet. Back pain is just the most inconvenient form of pain that typically forces people to acknowledge that they have a problem. If your leg hurts, you will probably shift your weight to the other side of your body, and then keep going. Back pain is much harder to ignore. Being forced to stop and take care of your back will force you to do other things that will benefit the rest of your body.

# Benefits Beyond the Back

Humans are really not designed for the amount of sitting and sedentary schedules that most of us have to keep. Our bodies are designed to be mobile for much of the day. Because you spend so much time sitting, all of your body suffers; it is just your back that is the most noticeable. As you age, the stiffness in your legs gets to be a lot more obvious if you try to sit for a couple of hours at a time. When you make a conscious effort to stand up at least once an hour, your legs will feel better, and it will take some of the tension out of your shoulders since you won't have them held in the unnatural position that you use to type.

I definitely recommend that you have a standing desk, if possible. However, you will still need to remember to move around at least once an hour. You absolutely need to give your arms a rest to avoid causing yourself upper back pain. Ailments like carpel tunnel are caused by too much repetition. By doing something else for a couple of minutes, going for a quick walk, or even just doing a bit of stretching, you are helping your entire body.

When you adopt a diet that focuses on anti-inflammatory foods, your other pains will start to be reduced as well. Because these diets are used primarily as a way of losing weight, you will have the added benefit of getting your weight under control. Since most of us who spend hours sitting at a desk have a bit of extra weight that we need to lose, losing weight can be beneficial to joints, as well as many other systems in the body. Eating is something that many cultures do without really giving the activity much thought. This leads to eating foods that are highly processed, lower in nutrients, and high in sugar. There is also a very unhealthy tendency to want to treat ourselves with junk food *because* we don't feel that we have time to eat any other treat. If we have to work late and didn't plan on it, we visit vending machines or order unhealthy foods to allow us to keep working. We grab a bag of chips at lunch time so that we can work an extra 30 minutes before taking lunch. We take one of the donuts from the breakroom after adding a mix of things to our coffee. All of this is incredibly unhealthy for your entire body, not just your back. It is just the warnings signs from your back that make you really notice how bad things have gotten. Unless you injure yourself doing strenuous activity, the odds are that your back pain stems from years of wear and tear that are caused by a less than optimal life style.

Back pain is really a symptom of something more seriously wrong in many cases. By opting to take medicine instead of changing your life style, you are just ignoring the real problems. Continuing to do the same things in the same way can not only do more damage to your back, but the rest of your body as well. As Chapters 9 and 10 point out, there are many activities and motions that can reduce the pain you experience, regardless of the initial cause of that pain. Even if you hurt your back while playing a sport, the changes to your diet will help reduce the pain.

Your back is literally the part of you that holds everything else together. Pain in your back is often accompanied by pain in other body parts. And sometimes, pain in other body parts is a sign of a problem with your back. Anything you do to promote a better life style for your back is going to benefit the rest of your body and your mind since you won't be obsessed with pain. As always, you will need to be careful with any new exercise routines you begin, and you should consult a physician before you get started. Don't use this as an excuse to keep putting it off though. Your entire body stands to benefit from a life style that is designed to help reduce or eliminate back pain, and so you should take a better course of action to prevent future problems.

# How Your Whole Body Can Benefit

The kinds of activities that you do for the benefit of your back will also benefit many other parts of your body. While many people say that you should sit up straight for your back, good posture helps all of the parts of your body. When you sit up straight, your arms are in a better position to type, putting less stress on your neck and shoulders. By holding your body even, your hips will have a more even distribution of its load. Although it seems counter-intuitive, even your legs and feet benefit from great posture. Good posture includes the way you position your legs. You should never cross your legs – that is bad for your entire body, but particularly for your back and legs. Don't sit with your legs spread wide apart either. Your legs should be at a 90-degree angle from your hips, and then your knees should be at a 90-degree angle. This ensures that no part of your body is under additional stress. Good posture is fully body positive (not to mention the benefit to your organs).

Exercise is obviously beneficial for your entire body, including joints, digestion, and circulatory systems. As I've said many times before, you have to be careful about the exercises you do. You not only have to be careful of your back, you have to take the rest of your body into account. Essentially, you have to go with the capabilities of your weakest area. Make sure that you work within your limitations so that you don't hurt yourself further. Getting accustomed to being careful of your back when you are working out will make it a lot easier to be more conscious of other potential health issues. By the time your back starts to hurt, there are probably other parts of your body that also need attention and care. If you have been putting taking care of them off, you need to be particularly careful of them when you start to exercise.

Increased awareness of your habits will help your entire body. Since many of the things you do to help your back benefit at least a couple of other parts of your body, correcting your bad habits will start to mend other problems that you may have been ignoring or that have not manifested themselves yet. It is past time to treat the problem, but now that you are working to do a better job of caring for your back, you will be much more likely to take other problems more seriously.

As you work to improve your habits, you will almost certainly notice other changes in your body. Changes to your exercise levels and diet helps your digestive track, which means you will better process your foods and become more regular. Getting down to a healthy weight reduces the amount of stress to your heart because it doesn't take as much work to move the blood through your body. Less weight on your legs means that your legs and hips will have less pressure on them.

Adopting a largely anti-inflammatory diet is ideal for anyone who has other painful conditions, such as arthritis or fibromyalgia. Your back pain may help you to start analyzing your diet more, but other regular pains probably already have you taking pain medications regularly. Arthritis is a particularly painful ailment that makes it difficult to complete regular activities. If you have broken some of your bones in the past, you will start to have reminders of that more often as you age. For all kinds of pain, an anti-inflammatory diet can reduce almost any kind of pain. Sure, it can be difficult in the beginning to give up certain foods, but in the end it is well worth it to have your pain reduced without having to take medications to do it.

All of these changes also affect your mental health. Depression and anxiety are tied to pain, and worrying about constant pain is a type of torture that affects the mind. You begin to try to anticipate pain or adopt unhealthy workarounds in your daily life, which hurts your mental health. Most of the medications affect your cognitive abilities as well, reducing how much you can do, which triggers anxiety over falling behind on your regular activities. Pain of any kind is something that most people cannot simply ignore. As you try to anticipate issues, you lose focus on other, more important things because you are afraid of hurting again. Healing your back and finding activities that facilitate a healthier life style offers you a peace of mind that you likely have not experienced since the pains began. Meditation is one of the best things you could do to help your mental health as well. Forcing yourself to take time out of your schedule to just focus on the current moment gives your brain a chance to rest. Meditation poses can vary based on your body's current abilities – you don't have to cross your legs and sit on the floor. You can meditate for a couple of minutes while you are at work when you start to get stressed. If you find that your workload is causing you to feel anxious, you are more likely to fall into bad habits, especially returning to the use of bad posture. Meditation can help you get better control over that anxiety while re-focusing on your posture. The act of meditating makes most people feel more relaxed, which will make it easier to assume better posture. Your mind and body are not two different things, but two different aspects of who you are. Taking care of your mental health will boost your ability to be healthier, and acting healthier will boost your mental abilities.

# Mind over Medicine

I definitely understand the need for medication. There are some kinds of pain and some situations when pain killers or relaxers are required – the problem is that we have become far too dependent on medication. The effects of that dependency ranges from tolerance (which means you have to take more pills to get the same level of pain relief) to addiction and death. None of those effects are good. And your body really was not designed for taking any kind of medication. Pills and tablets are most effective when you use them as an absolutely last resort, or the final option before surgery. There are very few cases when anyone should be recommended opioids, and a person taking opioids should be monitored as much as a patient who has just been through surgery. Those kinds of heavy drugs rarely have any place in a home, and should be kept to a hospital where the patient's use of them can be controlled. They are not comparable to over-the-counter medications. They really aren't comparable to most types of prescriptions. Opioids should only be used in the worst cases when the pain is so intense that the patient requires relief. No opioid should ever be allowed to be refilled without the patient returning to see a doctor. It is not a drug that treats the problem, and should never be used to mask the problem. If a person's pain is just as intense at the end of a short prescription of an opioid, that person needs a better treatment plan, not more opioids.

Even the use of over-the-counter medication is problematic. I do understand that some ailments will require a patient to take pills and tablets, but, again, it should not be the first thing that a person does to alleviate the pain. There are literally dozens of other things you can do to help manage the pain. Going out for a walk, meditating, and eating better do far more to resolve the pain *and* the problem. Even better, they do work for chronic pain and ailments that cause minor levels of pain daily.

The next time you start to feel pain in your back, take a minute to think about the pain and why you feel it. If your hands are hurting because of arthritis, maybe you need to take a break and relax for a few minutes. If you have sprained your ankle, don't reach for a pain killer. Instead, put a cold compress on your ankle to reduce your dependency on any medication. You may need some medication at some point following the sprain, but, honestly, taking a medication more than twice means you are probably constantly irritating the area because you are masking the pain and continuing to walk instead of giving your ankle a break. If your lower back and legs feel stiff after sleeping, you may need a new mattress. Don't take medication. Take a few minutes to analyze the problems so that you can avoid them in the future. Yes, I do know that this can be difficult. When I get a headache, my instinct is to reach for an over-the-counter solution, but over time, I have been fighting that automatic reaction. Instead of taking medicine for a couple of days to keep the pain at bay, I stand up and move around to give my shoulders a break. I have noticed that sitting at my desk for even an hour can start

# Mind over Medicine

I definitely understand the need for medication. There are some kinds of pain and some situations when pain killers or relaxers are required – the problem is that we have become far too dependent on medication. The effects of that dependency ranges from tolerance (which means you have to take more pills to get the same level of pain relief) to addiction and death. None of those effects are good. And your body really was not designed for taking any kind of medication. Pills and tablets are most effective when you use them as an absolutely last resort, or the final option before surgery. There are very few cases when anyone should be recommended opioids, and a person taking opioids should be monitored as much as a patient who has just been through surgery. Those kinds of heavy drugs rarely have any place in a home, and should be kept to a hospital where the patient's use of them can be controlled. They are not comparable to over-the-counter medications. They really aren't comparable to most types of prescriptions. Opioids should only be used in the worst cases when the pain is so intense that the patient requires relief. No opioid should ever be allowed to be refilled without the patient returning to see a doctor. It is not a drug that treats the problem, and should never be used to mask the problem. If a person's pain is just as intense at the end of a short prescription of an opioid, that person needs a better treatment plan, not more opioids.

Even the use of over-the-counter medication is problematic. I do understand that some ailments will require a patient to take pills and tablets, but, again, it should not be the first thing that a person does to alleviate the pain. There are literally dozens of other things you can do to help manage the pain. Going out for a walk, meditating, and eating better do far more to resolve the pain *and* the problem. Even better, they do work for chronic pain and ailments that cause minor levels of pain daily.

The next time you start to feel pain in your back, take a minute to think about the pain and why you feel it. If your hands are hurting because of arthritis, maybe you need to take a break and relax for a few minutes. If you have sprained your ankle, don't reach for a pain killer. Instead, put a cold compress on your ankle to reduce your dependency on any medication. You may need some medication at some point following the sprain, but, honestly, taking a medication more than twice means you are probably constantly irritating the area because you are masking the pain and continuing to walk instead of giving your ankle a break. If your lower back and legs feel stiff after sleeping, you may need a new mattress. Don't take medication. Take a few minutes to analyze the problems so that you can avoid them in the future. Yes, I do know that this can be difficult. When I get a headache, my instinct is to reach for an over-the-counter solution, but over time, I have been fighting that automatic reaction. Instead of taking medicine for a couple of days to keep the pain at bay, I stand up and move around to give my shoulders a break. I have noticed that sitting at my desk for even an hour can start to make my shoulders tense. It doesn't happen often, but the pain is telling me that I am doing something wrong.

Real healing requires you to understand and treat the problem. It is as much a psychological puzzle as it is a physical inconvenience. If your car starts to have problems, your reaction isn't to pump some new gas or oil into it and hope it helps. You go to a mechanic who can determine what is wrong (or if you are experienced in car repairs, you do it yourself). You then treat the problem. If you have a pain in your chest, you don't take pills and hope that the pain stops – you go to a doctor to find out the cause. If your leg hurts, you probably don't continue with your regular activities. In all of these situations, you look for a solution to the problem, and not just a band aid to cover it up. There is no medication that fixes back problems – all pain killers are different kinds of band aids. You need to find out what is wrong, then follow through with the correct treatment. In the beginning, it is going to be difficult, but that is part of what makes the natural solutions so appealing. As the pieces fall into place (the source of the pain, the triggers, and the solution), you will get a sense of accomplishment while helping your back to heal.

Changing a bad habit is not something that most people can easily do, but that is what really makes it rewarding. Refraining from taking medicine will be difficult in the beginning, but that is part of the necessary changes that you need to make. It is a matter of mind over medicine. The more you are able to do for yourself, the less reliant you will be on medicine. In the end, that is best for not only your back, but your entire body and your mind.

www.ingramcontent.com/pod-product-compliance
Lightning Source LLC
Chambersburg PA
CBHW071358210526
45465CB00001B/146